**W9-ADB-722**

*James R. Evans, PhD*
*Editor*

# Forensic Applications of QEEG and Neurotherapy

*Forensic Applications of QEEG and Neurotherapy* has been co-published simultaneously as *Journal of Neurotherapy*, Volume 9, Number 3, 2005.

*Pre-publication*
*REVIEWS,*
*COMMENTARIES,*
*EVALUATIONS . . .*

"Contains five studies and one review that highlight the utility of QEEG with regard to such topics as examination of lying and deception, individual differences in convicted murderers, and the effectiveness of neurotherapy within forensic populations. Though THE READER WILL FIND ALL CONTRIBUTIONS INTERESTING AND INFORMATIVE, the studies reported by authors Vendemia, Caine, and Evans is novel in it's approach. The findings point toward neurophysiological changes that may be resultant of various factors associated with long-term incarceration. The contribution of Thornton, in which a new nonverbal experimental design is employed to exam lie detection, is also particularly engaging. The findings from this study suggest differing patterns of regional activity that are associated with anxiety versus guilt."

**D. Erik Everhart, PhD**
*Associate Professor*
*Director*
*Program in Neuroscience*
*Department of Psychology*
*East Carolina University*

*More pre-publication*
*REVIEWS, COMMENTARIES, EVALUATIONS . . .*

" **A**N IMPORTANT CONTRIBU-
TION TO THE LITERATURE.
. . . A WELCOME ADDITION to any
reader interested in QEEG and neurotherapy."

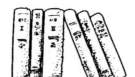

**David W. Harrison, PhD**
*Associate Professor and Director*
*Behavioral Neuroscience Laboratory*
*Virginia Tech*

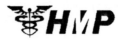 **HMP**

The Haworth Medical Press®
An Imprint of The Haworth Press, Inc.

# Forensic Applications of QEEG and Neurotherapy

*Forensic Applications of QEEG and Neurotherapy* has been co-published simultaneously as *Journal of Neurotherapy*, Volume 9, Number 3, 2005.

## Monographic Separates from the *Journal of Neurotherapy*

For additional information on these and other Haworth Press titles, including descriptions, tables of contents, reviews, and prices, use the QuickSearch catalog at http://www.HaworthPress.com.

*Forensic Applications of QEEG and Neurotherapy,* edited by James R. Evans, PhD (Vol. 9, No. 3, 2005) *Examines new and potentially very useful ways of verifying, preventing, and treating criminal behaviors; provides many valuable references for clinicians and researchers.*

*New Developments in Blood Flow Hemoencephalography,* edited by Tim Tinius, PhD (Vol. 8, No. 3, 2004) *Introduces the technique of operant conditioning of brain blood flow via feedback of information on oxygenation and brain temperature obtained by non-invasive instrumentation.*

*Quantitative Electroencephalographic Analysis (QEEG) Databases for Neurotherapy: Description, Validation, and Application,* edited by Joel F. Lubar, PhD (Vol. 7, No. 3/4, 2003) *Provides cutting-edge information on quantitative electroencephalographic analysis (QEEG), the most popular QEEG databases, and QEEG's applications in medicine.*

# Forensic Applications of QEEG and Neurotherapy

James R. Evans, PhD
Editor

*Forensic Applications of QEEG and Neurotherapy* has been co-published simultaneously as *Journal of Neurotherapy*, Volume 9, Number 3 2005.

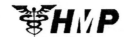

The Haworth Medical Press®
An Imprint of The Haworth Press, Inc.

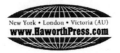

New York • London • Victoria (AU)
www.HaworthPress.com

Published by

The Haworth Medical Press®, 10 Alice Street, Binghamton, NY 13904-1580 USA

The Haworth Medical Press® is an imprint of The Haworth Press, Inc., 10 Alice Street, Binghamton, NY 13904-1580 USA.

*Forensic Applications of QEEG and Neurotherapy* has been co-published simultaneously as *Journal of Neurotherapy*, Volume 9, Number 3, 2005.

Cover design by Marylouise Doyle.

**Library of Congress Cataloging-in-Publication Data**

Forensic applications of QEEG and neurotherapy / James R. Evans, editor.
    p. ; cm.
    Simultaneously published as Journal of neurotherapy, volume 9, no. 3 2005.
    Includes bibliographical references and index.
    ISBN-13: 978-0-7890-3078-8 (hard cover : alk. paper)
    ISBN-10: 0-7890-3078-0 (hard cover : alk. paper)
    ISBN-13: 978-0-7890-3079-5 (soft cover : alk. paper)
    ISBN-10: 0-7890-3079-9 (soft cover : alk. paper)
    1. Electroencephalography. 2. Biofeedback training. 3. Medical jurisprudence. 4. Juvenile delinquency.
    [DNLM: 1. Electroencephalography–methods. 2. Biofeedback (Psychology) 3. Forensic Medicine–methods. 4. Juvenile Delinquency–prevention & control. 5. Juvenile Delinquency–psychology. WL 150 F715 2006] I. Evans, James R.
    RC386.6.E43F67 2006
    616.8′047547–dc22

                                 2006002579

# Indexing, Abstracting & Website/Internet Coverage

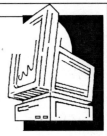

This section provides you with a list of major indexing & abstracting services and other tools for bibliographic access. That is to say, each service began covering this periodical during the year noted in the right column. Most Websites which are listed below have indicated that they will either post, disseminate, compile, archive, cite or alert their own Website users with research-based content from this work. (This list is as current as the copyright date of this publication.)

<u>Abstracting, Website/Indexing Coverage</u> . . . . . . . . <u>Year When Coverage Began</u>

- *Analgesia File, Dannemiller Memorial Education Foundation, Texas <http://www.pain.com>* . . . . . . . . . . . . . . . . . . . . . . . . . . . . 2003

- *Biology Digest (in print & online) <http://www.infotoday.com>* . . 2003

- *Business Source Corporate: coverage of nearly 3,350 quality magazines and journals; designed to meet the diverse information needs of corporations; EBSCO Publishing <http://www.epnet.com/corporate/bsourcecorp.asp>.* . . . . . . . . . . . . 2003

- *CINAHL (Cumulative Index to Nursing & Allied Health Literature), in print, EBSCO, and SilverPlatter, DataStar, and PaperChase. <http://www.cinahl.com>* . . . . . . . . . . . . . . . . 2005

- *EBSCOhost Electronic Journals Service (EJS) <http://ejournals.ebsco.com>.* . . . . . . . . . . . . . . . . . . . . . . . . . . 2001

- *Elsevier Scopus <http://www.info.scopus.com>* . . . . . . . . . . . . . . 2005

- *EMBASE.com (The Power of EMBASE + MEDLINE Combined) <http://www.embase.com>.* . . . . . . . . . . . . . . . . . . . . . . . . . . . . 2002

- *EMBASE/Excerpta Medica Secondary Publishing Division. Included in newsletters, review journals, major reference works, magazines and abstract journals <http://www.elsevier.nl>.* . . . . . . . . . . . . . . . . . . . . . . . . . . . . . . 2002

(continued)

(continued)

*Special Bibliographic Notes related to special journal issues (separates) and indexing/abstracting:*

- indexing/abstracting services in this list will also cover material in any "separate" that is co-published simultaneously with Haworth's special thematic journal issue or DocuSerial. Indexing/abstracting usually covers material at the article/chapter level.
- monographic co-editions are intended for either non-subscribers or libraries which intend to purchase a second copy for their circulating collections.
- monographic co-editions are reported to all jobbers/wholesalers/approval plans. The source journal is listed as the "series" to assist the prevention of duplicate purchasing in the same manner utilized for books-in-series.
- to facilitate user/access services all indexing/abstracting services are encouraged to utilize the co-indexing entry note indicated at the bottom of the first page of each article/chapter/contribution.
- this is intended to assist a library user of any reference tool (whether print, electronic, online, or CD-ROM) to locate the monographic version if the library has purchased this version but not a subscription to the source journal.
- individual articles/chapters in any Haworth publication are also available through the Haworth Document Delivery Service (HDDS).

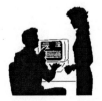

# Forensic Applications of QEEG and Neurotherapy

## CONTENTS

## ABOUT THE EDITOR

**James R. Evans, PhD,** is Professor Emeritus at the University of South Carolina. He is retired from teaching in the Psychology Department. A licensed clinical and school psychologist, he has a private practice in Greenville, South Carolina. He has been active in the fields of quantitative EEG and neurofeedback, both as a clinical practitioner and researcher. Dr. Evans is BCIA–Certified in neurotherapy, is certified as a QEEG technologist and has Fellow status in the International Society of Neuronal Regulation. He is a frequent contributor to the *Journal of Neurotherapy*.

# Preface

## OUR THIRD SPECIAL ISSUE

*It was the best of times; it was the worst of times.* According to the U.S. Department of Justice we live in the worst of times. For 50 years between 1925 and 1975, the incarceration rate in this country hovered around one-tenth of a percent, with an occasional blip during wartime or economic strife. As recently as 1968 only 95 of every 100,000 citizens were in prison (Vogel, 2003). But our incarceration rate is currently five times higher, 486 per 100,000 adults, and when juvenile and other facilities are taken into account more than 2.25 million Americans are now behind bars (Harrison & Beck, 2004). The U.S. accounts for nearly a quarter of an estimated 9 million people in penal institutions throughout the world. Only the nations of Belarus, Kazakhstan, Turkmenistan, and the Russian Federation lock up their citizens as frequently as America does (Walmsley, 2003). Federal prisons are operating at 40% above capacity while other industrialized nations seem to live in the sleepy past, with incarceration rates matching ours of a half-century ago: 116 per 100,000 in Canada, 91 and 85 in Germany and France, and 53 in Japan. Some say Rome fell because taxes were too high. In future history books will they write that America fell because its prisons were too full? Either our culture has become five to ten times more dangerous or coarse in the last quarter-century, or we are witnessing a crisis in law enforcement.

Change in the law is slow but constant. Law continually absorbs new technology and new models of human nature. Today behavioral and cognitive neuroscience are on the verge of retooling many of the concepts underlying criminal responsibility. Legal tests for mental incapac-

[Haworth co-indexing entry note]: "Preface." Kaiser, David A. Co-published simultaneously in *Journal of Neurotherapy* (The Haworth Medical Press, an imprint of The Haworth Press, Inc.) Vol. 9, No. 3, 2005, pp. xxi-xxii; and: *Forensic Applications of QEEG and Neurotherapy* (ed: James R. Evans) The Haworth Medical Press, an imprint of The Haworth Press, Inc., 2005, pp. xiii-xiv. Single or multiple copies of this article are available for a fee from The Haworth Document Delivery Service [1-800-HAWORTH, 9:00 a.m. - 5:00 p.m. (EST). E-mail address: docdelivery@haworthpress. com].

ity, culpability, willfulness, and premeditation may be redrawn as advances in electroencephalography and neuroimaging techniques mount in the coming years. As our understanding of biophysical causes of human misbehavior increases, criminal rehabilitation will necessarily improve. Clinical neuroscience, of which neurotherapy plays an essential role, may help reverse the worst-of-times trend of the last quarter-century through assessment, prevention, and treatment of antisocial and violent tendencies, as well as addressing drug addiction. Between 1984 and 1996 California built 21 new prisons and only one new university (Ambrosio & Schiraldi, 1997). This is a trend which must be reversed if America is to survive as a free and independent nation deep into this century.

What follows is the third special issue of the *Journal of Neurotherapy* and the first issue which I have had the privilege to edit. Congratulations to Jim Evans, who developed the issue and guided every author's contribution, and to Editors Tim Tinius and David Trudeau and Managing Editor Darlene Nelson for their tremendous efforts in moving it all towards completion. Learning to behave is not as easy as parents would hope or ethics professors might make it out to be. For this reason we have law, an ancient and ongoing experiment in behavioral regulation between strangers or acquaintances based on centralized (governmental) conflict resolution and revenge. More importantly, it is grounded in our self-knowledge. As the human mind becomes transparent to science and gives up its secrets one by one, the law will surely benefit and we may see the best of times. . . . or perhaps, again, the worst of times.

*David A. Kaiser, PhD*
*Rochester Institute of Technology*
*18 Lomb Memorial Drive*
*Rochester, NY 14625*

## REFERENCES

Ambrosio, T., & Schiraldi, V. (1997). *Trends in state spending, 1987-1995*. Washington, DC: The Justice Policy Institute.

Harrison, P. M., & Beck, A. J. (2004). *Prisoners in 2004* (Bulletin NCJ 210677). Washington, DC: US Department of Justice.

Vogel, R. D. (2003). Capitalism and incarceration revisited. *Monthly Review, 55*, 38-55.

Walmsley, R. (2003). *World prison population list*. London: Home Office Research, Development and Statistics Directorate.

# Introduction:
# Forensic Applications
# of QEEG and Neurotherapy

James R. Evans, PhD

Many of us who have followed the field of neurotherapy from its beginnings have long believed that forensic settings would be ideal locations for this form of treatment. After all, there is a very high incidence of attention deficit hyperactivity disorder and related symptoms among persons convicted of crimes and a great many criminal acts involve impulsive behaviors or loss of control of emotions such as rage. Improved control of behavior and emotion are among the most commonly reported results of neurotherapeutic treatment. Research and clinical experience also demonstrate positive effects of neurotherapy with alcohol and drug abuse and depression, both common accompaniments of criminal behaviors. Furthermore, incarcerated persons would be available for treatment sessions over extended periods of time and can be given strong incentives for successful participation, such as "good behavior" credit toward early release. Why then have there been so few research and clinical neurotherapy applications in forensic settings?

In the early 1990s this editor made several attempts to develop a neurotherapy program in his home state. Initially these attempts re-

James R. Evans is Professor Emeritus at the University of South Carolina, and has a private practice in Greenville, SC.

Address correspondence to: James R. Evans, PhD, 183 Morning Lake Drive, Moore, SC 29369.

[Haworth co-indexing entry note]: "Introduction: Forensic Applications of QEEG and Neurotherapy." Evans, James R. Co-published simultaneously in *Journal of Neurotherapy* (The Haworth Medical Press, an imprint of The Haworth Press, Inc.) Vol. 9, No. 3, 2005, pp. 1-3; and: *Forensic Applications of QEEG and Neurotherapy* (ed: James R. Evans) The Haworth Medical Press, an imprint of The Haworth Press, Inc., 2005, pp. 1-3. Single or multiple copies of this article are available for a fee from The Haworth Document Delivery Service [1-800-HAWORTH, 9:00 a.m. - 5:00 p.m. (EST). E-mail address: docdelivery@haworthpress.com].

Available online at http://www.haworthpress.com/web/JN
© 2005 by The Haworth Press, Inc. All rights reserved.
doi:10.1300/J184v09n03_01

ceived a lukewarm reception but by the middle of the decade a shift in philosophy from rehabilitation to punishment in the penal system occurred and it became obvious that no such program was to be. Perhaps this shift also occurred elsewhere, or maybe a punishment philosophy has always existed in many places. In any event it seems most leaders of the forensic community are not yet ready for neurotherapy. One can hope, however, that this situation is changing, however slowly, and that as more research findings supporting its efficacy are published it will become a major force in both prevention and treatment of criminal behaviors.

This volume contains reports on two of the very few studies known to exist in which neurotherapy was used in forensic settings where attempts were made to measure outcome. Although the studies by Smith and Sams and Martin and Johnson contain some shortcomings in terms of experimental design, both provide support for the efficacy of neurotherapy in such settings and will hopefully provide impetus for much more related research involving sophisticated design, and larger numbers of participants from diverse groups.

As important as treatment and rehabilitation of offenders may be, prevention of criminal behaviors may be even more important. Here again, neurotherapy can play a major role through early treatment intervention with persons at risk for criminal behavior, such as those with behavioral or neurological conditions associated with sociopathology or impulsivity. Attention deficit hyperactivity disorder, especially hyperactive-impulsive and mixed types, intermittent explosive disorder and oppositional defiant disorder are three disorders which come to mind but any disorder of executive function would qualify. Accurate and early diagnosis of the predisposing conditions and their physiological cause is important, and it is here that quantified EEG (QEEG) measures are especially useful. A growing body of research supports the value of QEEG findings in delineating abnormalities of brain electrical activity related to problems with executive control, including engaging in violent acts. Furthermore, many neurotherapy practitioners rely on QEEG results to help plan specific treatment protocols. QEEG research with death row inmates by Vendemia, Caine, and Evans reported in this issue adds to existing research supporting cortical dysfunction in frontal areas in many persons convicted of violent acts. While there is strong evidence for neurobiological abnormalities among criminals, there is evidence that external environmental factors can also play major roles separately or in interaction with abnormal neurology. The article by Kaiser emphasizes this, as he provides evidence supporting the role of large group size and related feelings of anonymity and rejection to school violence by teens.

Children and adults who have difficulty sustaining attention and controlling impulses often struggle with interpersonal relationships, not only with parents, teachers and spouses, but with law enforcement personnel as well. Such difficulties may lead to seeking relationships with individuals or groups where affiliation needs are taken advantage of, such as by gang leaders who use these vulnerable individuals in criminal dealings. Similarly, these individuals may also be predisposed to impulsive but false confessions to crimes or may fail to attend appropriately to directions from police, judges and others in forensic settings, which could lead to a high incidence of such persons inappropriately convicted of crimes. Highly reliable and valid measures of deception would be extremely useful in such cases, as present methods of lie detection are considered insufficiently reliable to be used as evidence in court. Articles by Thornton and by Vendemia, Buzan, Green, and Schillaci in this special issue describe sophisticated QEEG measures of deception which could revolutionize this aspect of forensics.

It is the hope of this editor that the research and speculation reported here portends later forensic editions a few years from now which will contain articles providing strong scientific support for the value of neurotherapy and QEEG in preventing, diagnosing, and treating forensic-related issues.

# SCIENTIFIC ARTICLES

# Quantitative EEG Findings in Convicted Murderers

Jennifer M. C. Vendemia, PhD
Kelly E. Caine, BA
James R. Evans, PhD

**SUMMARY.** In this study we examined the QEEGs of convicted murderers ($n = 73$) living on death row, referred by attorneys, and compared them to a control group ($n = 23$) referred for neuropsychological evaluation by physicians, attorneys, or a State Vocational Rehabilitation Department. The individuals living on death row committed murders

Jennifer M. C. Vendemia is affiliated with the Department of Psychology, University of South Carolina.

Kelly E. Caine is affiliated with the Human Factors and Aging Lab, Georgia Institute of Technology.

James R. Evans is Professor Emeritus of Psychology, University of South Carolina.

Address correspondence to: Jennifer M. C. Vendemia, University of South Carolina, Department of Psychology, Columbia, SC 29208 (E-mail: Vendemia@mindspring.com).

[Haworth co-indexing entry note]: "Quantitative EEG Findings in Convicted Murderers." Vendemia, Jennifer M. C., Kelly E. Caine, and James R. Evans. Co-published simultaneously in *Journal of Neurotherapy* (The Haworth Medical Press, an imprint of The Haworth Press, Inc.) Vol. 9, No. 3, 2005, pp. 5-29; and: *Forensic Applications of QEEG and Neurotherapy* (ed: James R. Evans) The Haworth Medical Press, an imprint of The Haworth Press, Inc., 2005, pp. 5-29. Single or multiple copies of this article are available for a fee from The Haworth Document Delivery Service [1-800-HAWORTH, 9:00 a.m. - 5:00 p.m. (EST). E-mail address: docdelivery@haworthpress.com].

Available online at http://www.haworthpress.com/web/JN
doi:10.1300/J184v09n03_02

during robberies, drug deals, rapes, and crimes of passion. They all had
suspected or known histories of traumatic brain injury; some had comor-
bidities of schizophrenia, depression, and other psychiatric diagnoses.
The individuals in the control group had a history of head trauma resulting primarily from motor vehicle accidents; a few had the comorbidity
of depression. The murderers were randomly divided into two separate
groups for comparisons with the control group. Coherence (within
broad-band alpha) scores were calculated between all scalp electrode
sites and fast-fourier spectral analyses were performed for each channel
for two QEEG samples of at least 60 seconds (after artifact removal) recorded during eyes-closed. Spatial principal components derived from
the mean peak-to-peak magnitude were calculated for several bands of
EEG and submitted to 2 × 2 (death penalty × handedness) ANOVAs.
Murderers had reduced mean peak-to-peak magnitude across all bands
similar to that seen in broad spectrum EEG studies of aging. At anterior
regions murderers had reduced high theta and high alpha suggesting impaired attention. There was significantly higher coherence in controls in
the alpha range between and among central and posterior sites. These
findings are used to support the theory that time on death row facilitates
"cognitive aging." *[Article copies available for a fee from The Haworth Document Delivery Service: 1-800-HAWORTH. E-mail address: <docdelivery@
haworthpress.com> Website: <http://www.HaworthPress.com> © 2005 by The
Haworth Press, Inc. All rights reserved.]*

**KEYWORDS.** QEEG, cognitive impairment, murderers, death row, aging

## INTRODUCTION

The number of murderers living on death row and the amount of time
they spend on death row has been increasing steadily since the revision
of state capital punishment laws in 1976. Many studies have reported
brain abnormalities in individuals convicted of murder, and these abnormalities may be exacerbated by the pattern of cognitive and physical
decline documented in individuals who endure incarceration on death
row (Johnson, 1979). In the only published quantitative EEG (QEEG)
study of individuals on death row, Evans and Park (1997) compared the
QEEG of such incarcerated individuals to established norms and found
several significant differences. Although focal brain damage and cognitive impairment are highly correlated with violent crime and murder,
they are not predictive. The current study attempted to extend previous

QEEG findings and to separate pre-existing focal brain damage from pathology related to death row by comparing two groups of individuals serving time on death row to a group of matched controls.

Evidence in the literature suggests that violent offenders very frequently have brain abnormalities (for review and meta-analysis, see Cunningham & Vigen, 2002). In eight studies reporting the neurological impairments of individuals on death row, three identified minor or major neurological impairments in 33 to 75% of cases (Freedman & Hemenway, 2000; Lewis, Pincus, Feldman, Jackson, & Bard, 1986; Lewis et al., 1988); four identified head trauma in 24 to 100% of the cases (Freedman & Hemenway, 2000; Frierson, Schwartz-Watts, Morgan, & Malone, 1998; Lewis et al., 1988, Lewis et al., 1986) and five identified abnormal EEG or PET scans in 50 to 100% of cases (Evans & Park, 1997; Frierson et al., 1998; Raine, Buchsbaum, & LaCasse, 1997; Raine et al., 1994; Raine et al., 1998).

Evans and Park (1997) compared the QEEG of 20 murderers to norms set in the Thatcher Life Span EEG Reference Database (Thatcher, Walker, & Guidice, 1987) for coherence (i.e., similarity of waveforms), phase (i.e., neural conduction time), and amplitude asymmetry (i.e., asymmetry of wave amplitude) in delta, theta, alpha, and beta frequency bands. In twelve subjects they found coherence abnormalities involving any right frontal site (Fp2, F4, F8) and any right posterior site (P4, T6, O2). In murderers they found more right hemisphere phase abnormalities than left hemisphere phase abnormalities and a majority of phase abnormalities in the anterior regions. Twelve subjects had one or more amplitude asymmetries between F8 and T4, and 15 subjects had abnormally increased coherence.

A PET study comparing 41 murderers pleading not guilty by reason of insanity to 41 controls found reduced glucose metabolism in prefrontal cortex, superior parietal cortex, left angular gyrus, and the corpus callosum (Raine et al., 1997). A second PET study comparing nine affective (murder without premeditation) murderers to matched controls found a pattern of lower prefrontal activity and higher subcortical activity in murderers (Raine et al., 1998).

However, pre-existing brain abnormalities may only partially explain the locus and frequency of cortical abnormalities among death row inmates. Death row has been characterized as an extremely stressful environment. There is the stress of impending execution (Bluestone & McGahee, 1962); there are stressors based on the community dynamics with prisoners not serving time on death row as well as with guards (Arrigo & Fowler, 2001; Cunningham & Vigen, 2002), and there are physical stressors resulting from substandard living conditions (Cunningham & Vigen, 2002). Time spent on death row is associated with a cluster of psychological factors which some researchers believe may lead to "personality deterioration or actual insanity" (Johnson, 1979). These psychological symptoms include: (a) a sense of helplessness and defeat, (b) a sense of widespread and diffuse danger, (c) a perception of helpless vulnerability, (d) emotional emptiness, (e) loneliness and a deadening of feelings, and (f) a decline in mental and physical acuity. Lengthy stays on death row can exacerbate these symptoms (Gallermore & Panton, 1972).

Due to changing conditions in the justice system, inmates are enduring more time on death row which may lead to even greater changes in psychological state. Since the revision of state capital punishment laws in 1976 the number of inmates on death row has increased significantly while the number of inmates executed annually has remained constant (see Figure 1). This pair of trends has resulted in a growing population of inmates living on death row. In 2002, inmates were spending an average of 8.64 years on death row ($SDx = 5.79$). This was up from 1992 when inmates were spending an average of 6.31 years on death row ($SDx = 3.63$; U.S. Department of Justice, 2004).

FIGURE 1. Trends for prisoners on death row and the number of executions in the period from 1930 until 2002 (based on National Archive of Criminal Justice Data).

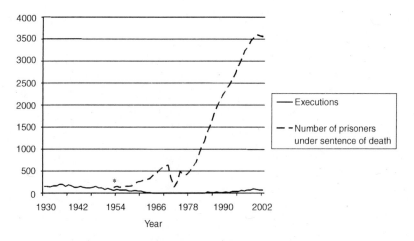

Year

*Number of prisoners under sentence of death unavailable for period before 1953.

The combination of brain abnormalities of violent offenders and the psychological consequences of spending time on death row may have a serious impact on mental status. The deterioration of mental acuities has been found to include drowsiness, listlessness, mental slowness, confusion, and forgetfulness (Johnson, 1979). These factors related to spending time on death row may impact the EEG. For example, cognitive decline may impact broad band beta, as a decrease in broad band beta power has been reported in normal aging subjects experiencing cognitive decline (Williamson et al., 1990). A similar trend has been observed in broad band alpha (Soininen et al., 1991). Perhaps also relevant are the findings of Adler, Bramesfeld, and Jajcevic (1999) who reported an increase in absolute power in the delta and theta bands in depressed subjects with mild cognitive impairments.

Broad band EEG can be subdivided into narrow bands that have been associated with specific cognitive activities. For example, broad band theta can be differentiated into two discrete bands associated with unique types of mental activity (for review, see Schacter, 1977). Increased low theta (4-5.45 Hz) activity correlates with decreased arousal and increased drowsiness, while high theta (6-7.45 Hz) activity correlates with increased attention and cognitive load. High theta normally is enhanced during tasks involving working memory (Klimesch, 1996) and has been associated with focused cognitive activities (Inouye, Ishihara, Shinosaki, Toi & Ukai, 1988; Ishihara & Yoshi, 1972; Mizuki, Kajimura, Kaie, Suetsuigi, 1992; Ramos, Corsi-Cabrera, Guevara, & Arce, 1993).

We hypothesized that as low theta is negatively correlated with arousal such as that produced during states of anxiety, individuals serving time on death row would produce less low theta than matched controls would produce. As high theta is positively correlated with cognitive activities, individuals on death row with minimal intellectual stimulation would produce less high theta than matched controls would produce.

Within the broad band alpha range, factor analytic work indicates discrete alpha frequency bands (Hermann & Schaerer, 1986; Mecklinger, Kramer, & Strayer, 1992). Individuals who self-reported poor sustained attentional abilities generated significantly more low alpha spectral magnitude than did high sustained attention subjects while performing tracking or decision making tasks; mid and high alpha bands did not discriminate (Crawford, Knebel, Vendemia, Kaplan, & Ratcliff, 1995). High sustained attention individuals have been found to generate more high alpha compared to low sustained attention individuals (Crawford, Clark, & Kitner-Triolo, 1996).

Because individuals on death row report drowsiness, listlessness and mental slowness (Gallermore & Panton, 1972), we predicted that they would generate more low alpha than matched controls would generate. Additionally, as individuals on death row report impaired cognitive abilities, perhaps related to impaired attention, it was expected that individuals on death row would have decreased high alpha when compared to matched controls.

Broad band beta activity can also be subdivided into discrete subbands. Low beta activity in the 11-15 Hz (beta-13) range has been associated with visual tracking (Mann, Sterman, & Kaiser, 1996), and beta activity in the 16-24 Hz (beta-16) range has been associated with enhanced attentional processing (Crawford et al., 1996; Crawford et al., 1995). Beta 16 also has been correlated with vigilance in individuals with more sustained attentional abilities (Crawford et al., 1996; Crawford et al., 1995). As observed in studies of cognitive impairment and depression, it was expected that participants on death row would generate less beta-13 and beta-16 compared to matched controls.

In the current study we examined the QEEGs of seventy-three individuals convicted of murder, who at the time of their evaluation were living on death row. Based on the work of Raine and colleagues (Raine et al., 1997, Raine et al., 1994, Raine et al., 1998, see discussion below) we compared their QEEGs to those of a control group of neurologically impaired, matched controls. We examined two classes of dependent variables: (a) mean peak-to-peak magnitude within low theta (3.5-5.45 Hz), high theta (5.5-7.45 Hz), low alpha (7.5-8.45 Hz), mid alpha (8.5-11.45 Hz), high alpha (11.5-13.45 Hz), beta-13 (13.5-16.45 Hz), and beta-16 (16.5-19.45 Hz) bands; and (b) coherence within broad band alpha (7.5-13.45 Hz).

Patterns of mean peak-to-peak power across electrode sites and coherence between electrode sites were explored using principal components analysis followed by statistical tests of the hypotheses. This strategy allows one to identify regions of patterns activation, and to test those patterns specifically. Several researchers have advocated the use of multivariate statistics in the exploration of EEG data due to the multivariate nature of the data as well as the applicability of these types of results to neurophysiological models of cognition (Barceló & Gale, 1997; Barceló, Gale, & Hall, 1995; Tucker & Roth, 1984). Reducing the dimensionality of an EEG dataset with principal components and then testing hypotheses is specifically suggested (Barceló & Gale, 1997; Duffy, Bartels, & Neff, 1986).

Patterns of coherence were predicted to discriminate death row inmates and matched controls. Evans and Park (1997) hypothesized that the observed patterns of increased coherence were related to decreased cortical differentiation. Based on these findings we expected that individuals serving time on death row would have abnormalities of increased coherence when compared with the control group. Additionally, based on Evans and Park (1997), we predicted that individuals serving time on death row would have more abnormalities of coherence in the right hemisphere than in the left hemisphere and more abnormalities involving coupling between relatively distant electrode sites (Fp1, Fp2, F3, F4, F7, or F8 to P3, P4, T5, T6, O1, or O2).

## *METHOD*

### *Participants*

The participants were selected from an archival data set from 10 years of neuropsychological evaluations. The overall set was divided into two groups of murderers based on date of collection and then separately compared to a single control group. Murderers in both groups ($n =$ 46 and $n = 27$) were referred by attorneys. The ages of murderers in group 1 ranged from 19 to 53 ($Mx = 30.67$, $Sdx = 8.62$), and the ages of those in group 2 ranged from 19 to 52 ($Mx = 32.00$, $Sdx = 9.54$). The mean age of murderers in both groups was lower than the mean age of all individuals on death rows in 2002 ($Mx = 39.00$; Bonczar & Snell, 2003). All participants in this study were male, and this matches the overall demographic of prisoners on death row (male = 98.6%, female = 1.4%; Bonczar & Snell, 2003). Fifty-four percent of all inmates under sentence of death in 2002 were Caucasian, 44% were African-American, 12% were Hispanic, and 2% fit other categories (Bonczar & Snell, 2003), while 64% of the current sample were Caucasian and 36% were African-American. The median educational level of inmates in groups 1 and 2 was 10.15 and 10.68, respectively. This was slightly lower than the median educational level of 11th grade for all inmates on death row in 2002 (Bonczar & Snell, 2003). The murders in this study were convicted of crimes including robbery, drug deals, rape, and crimes of passion; they met the definition proposed by Raine et al. (1994) of affective murderers. Report data for time spent on death row was available for a subset of 26 inmates. These inmates spent between 2 years and 16 years, four months on death row ($Mx = 3381$ days, $SDx = 1269$ days).

The control group participants ($n = 23$) were referred by physicians, attorneys, or a State Vocational Rehabilitation Department. The decision to use a neuropsychologically impaired control group was based on PET studies of murderers (Raine et al., 1997; Raine et al., 1994; Raine et al., 1998), and a recommendation in Evans and Park (1997). In this research, the control group was matched on a variety of demographic characteristics. Although there has been some debate regarding appropriate controls for murderers (i.e., Ladds & Trachtenburg, 1995), most researchers advocate the strategy of matching on brain trauma and psychiatric illness when studying murderers. As can be seen from Table 1, the control group did not significantly differ from either group of murderers in age, IQ or handedness. However, the control group did have a slightly higher education level [$t(67) = 2.11, p = .001$].

Reading level and arithmetic level (standard scores) results from the Wide Range Achievement Test (WRAT-R; Jastak & Wilkinson, 1984 or WRAT-3; Wilkinson, 1993) were not significantly different for murderers and controls, $t(43) = -.85, p = .20, t(21) = -.11, p = .91$. The means and standard deviations are given in Table 1. Scores for both groups were below average.

TABLE 1. Demographic Variables for Murderers on Death Row in Groups 1 and 2, as well as the Matched Control Group.

| Group | AGE | IQ | Education | Hand R | Hand L | WRAT (Standard Score) Reading | WRAT (Standard Score) Arithmetic |
|---|---|---|---|---|---|---|---|
| Study 1: Murderers (n = 46) | | | | 33 | 13 | | |
| M (SD) | 30.67 (8.62) | 91.83 (15.13) | 10.15 (1.86) | | | 88.17 (17.64) | 83.17 (15.79) |
| Study 2: Murderers (n = 27) | | | | 21 | 6 | | |
| M (SD) | 32.00 (9.54) | 92.96 (12.81) | 10.68 (2.44) | | | * | * |
| Control Group (n = 23) | | | | 14 | 9 | | |
| M (SD) | 40.00 (14.31) | 91.8 (16.28) | 12.26 (3.06) | | | 84.39 (17.04) | 78.50 (12.77) |
| Total (N = 96) | | | | 68 | 28 | | |
| M (SD) | 34.22 (10.82) | 92.20 (14.74) | 11.03 (2.45) | | | 85.65 (17.21) | 82.83 (13.53) |

*Data unavailable.

## Procedure

EEG was recorded with a Lexicor Medical Technologies Neuro-search-24 system (Lexicor Technologies, Boulder, CO) from anterior frontal (Fp1, Fp2), medial frontal (F3, F4), lateral frontal (F7, F8), central, (C3, C4), anterior temporal (T3, T4), posterior temporal (T5, T6), parietal (P3, P4), occipital (O1, O2), and midline (Fz, Cz, Pz) sites according to the international 10-20 system (Jasper, 1958) using an appropriately sized electrode cap (Electro-Cap International, Inc., Eaton, OH). Reference was to linked earlobes (A1, A2). Resistance was kept below 5000 ohms. EEG signals between 1 and 32 Hz were amplified with a gain setting of 32K. The sampling rate was 128 samples per second. A 60 Hz notch filter was used to reduce electrical noise.

Three minutes of EEG activity was sampled during an eyes-closed resting condition while participants sat in an upright position and asked to relax, to sit as still as possible, and to try to keep eyes closed and still. Data collection was initiated when each participant's raw EEG indicated eye and other movement artifacts were as minimal as deemed possible.

Recordings of the individuals convicted of murder were completed in rooms on "death rows" over a 10-year period, while recordings of matched controls were conducted in clinicians' offices over the same period.

## Data Analyses

EEG data were screened for artifact before conversion into Neuroscan format (Neuroscan Inc., Palo Alto, NM). Fast-fourier spectral analyses were performed for each channel (1-32 Hz) and mean magnitude was calculated for the following frequencies: low-theta (3.5-5.45 Hz), high-theta (5.5-7.45 Hz), low-alpha (7.5-8.45 Hz), mid-alpha (8.5-11.45 Hz), high-alpha (11.5-13.45 Hz), beta-13 (13.5-16.45 Hz), and beta-16 (16.5-19.45 Hz). Data were log transformed due to the commonly observed positively skewed frequency distribution of EEG with high kurtosis (Sterman, Mann, Kaiser, & Suyenobu, 1994).

## RESULTS

### Narrow Band Frequency Analyses

Principal components analysis with varimax rotation was run for each of the frequency bands across the 19 channels of data. Principal components allows for the extraction of related variance across electrode sites. When more than one effect occurs within a band, these effects can be evaluated separately. Additionally, variance not related to any specific component can be eliminated from further analysis.

The principal components from each band were individually submitted to 2 × 2 (group × handedness) ANOVAs. Component loadings were evaluated to localize effects across specific electrode sites on the scalp. Correlations were performed between the components and the demographic variables of IQ, age, and education.

We hypothesized that time spent on death row would impact components associated with the low and high theta as well as the low and high alpha. In order to test this hypothesis, we calculated correlations between the components and the number of days spent on death row for the subset of 26 death row inmates for whom we had these data.

### Death Row Group 1

*Low-Theta (3.5-5.45 Hz).* Two components accounted for 90.16% of the variance in low-theta scores. The first component had the strongest loadings on activity in the frontal regions (Fp1, Fp2, Fz, F3, F4, F7, F8), while the second component had the strongest loadings on activity in the parietal and occipital regions (P3, P4, O1, O2). A 2 × 2 (group × handedness) ANOVA revealed no significant differences between groups for either component. Figure 2 shows mean low theta activity in convicted murderers and neurologically impaired matched controls. There was a significant negative correlation between the first low theta component and age ($r = -.335, p = .005$), and a trend toward a significant positive correlation between the second low theta component and education ($r = .232, p = .055$). In the subset of inmates for whom time spent on death row was available ($n = 26$), there was a significant correlation between the second low theta component and time spent on death row such that individuals who had spent longer on death row generated more low theta in parietal and occipital regions ($r = .411, p = .018$).

*High-Theta (5.5-7.45 Hz).* A single component with loadings in frontal and parietal regions (Fp1, Fp2, Fz, F3, F4, Pz, P3, P4) explained 87.39% of the variance in high-theta activity. A 2 × 2 (group × handedness) ANOVA revealed a main effect for group, $F(1, 69) = 6.27, p = .015$, such that convicted murderers generated less high-theta compared to controls. Additionally, there was an interaction between group and handedness such that left-handed controls generated the most high-theta, followed by right-handed controls, then by right-handed con-

FIGURE 2. Mean log transformed magnitude of EEG in sub-bands of theta, alpha, and beta in individuals in Group 1 who received the death penalty and matched controls.

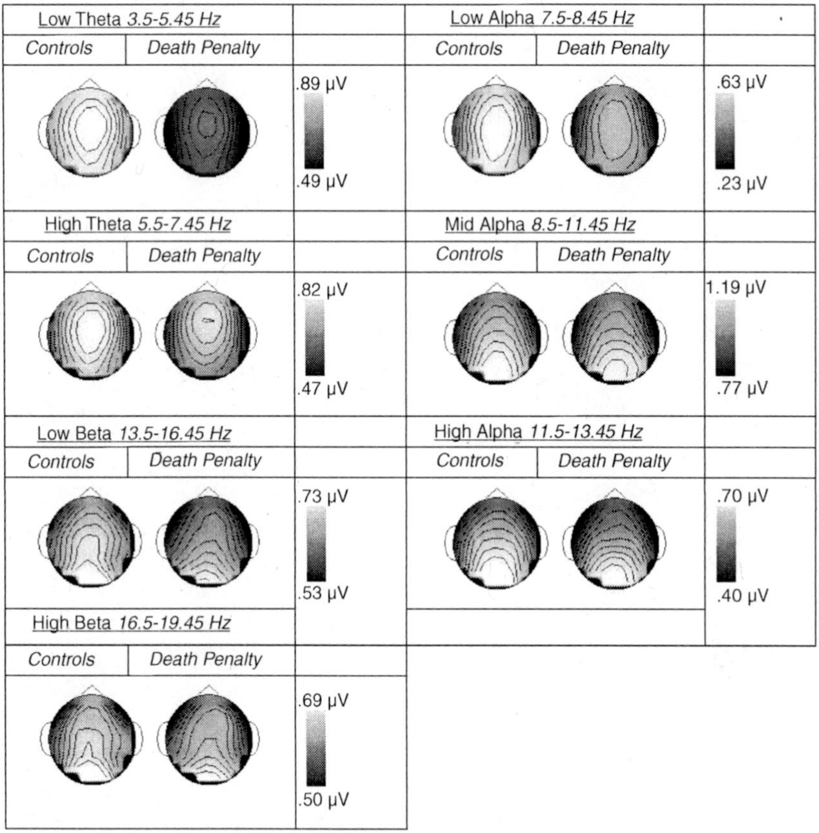

victed murderers, and then left-handed convicted murderers, $F(1, 69) = 4.34$, $p = .041$. Figure 2 shows mean high theta magnitude in convicted murderers and controls. There was a significant positive correlation between high-theta component and education ($r = .260$, $p = .031$).

*Low-Alpha (7.5-8.45 Hz).* A single component with loadings in the frontal and central regions (Fp1, Fp2, Fz, F3, F4, Cz, C3, C4) explained 91.90% of the variance in low-alpha activity. A 2 × 2 (group × handedness) ANOVA revealed a main effect for group such that convicted murderers had much lower scores on this component than controls, $F(1,$

69) = 9.97, $p$ = .002. Figure 2 shows mean low alpha magnitude in convicted murderers and controls. There was also a significant interaction, $F(1, 69)$ = 5.89, $p$ = .03. Left-handed controls scored the highest on the low alpha component, followed by right-handed controls, then right-handed individuals convicted murderers, and finally left-handed convicted murderers. There were no significant correlations between the low-alpha component and demographic data.

*Mid-Alpha (8.5-11.45 Hz).* A single component explained 91.90% of the variance in mid-alpha activity. A 2 × 2 (group × handedness) ANOVA revealed no significant effects. Figure 2 shows mean mid-alpha magnitude in murderers and controls. There was a significant negative correlation between the mid-alpha component and age ($r$ = −.286, $p$ = .017); younger individuals tended to have higher scores on this component than older individuals.

*High-Alpha (11.5-13.45 Hz).* Two components explained 90.71% of the variance in the high-alpha band. The first component loaded most strongly in the frontal and central regions (Fz, FP1, FP2, F3, F7, F8, C3, C4) while the second component loaded most strongly in the parietal and temporal regions (P3, P4, T3, T4, T5, T6). A 2 × 2 (group × handedness) ANOVA showed that controls had much higher scores on the first component than murderers, $F(1, 69)$ = 4.63, $p$ = .035. No significant differences were identified for the second high-alpha component. Figure 2 shows mean high-alpha magnitude in convicted murderers and controls. There was a trend towards a negative correlation between age and the second high-alpha component such that older individuals had lower scores on this component compared to younger individuals ($r$ = −.223, $p$ = .065).

*Beta-13 Activity (13.5-16.45 Hz).* Two components explained 87.91% of the variance in the Beta-13 band. The first component loaded most strongly in the parietal, occipital, and posterior temporal region (P3, P4, O1, O2, T5, T6), while the second component loaded most strongly in the frontal and central regions (FZ, FP1, FP2, F3, F7, F8, C3, C4). A 2 × 2 (group × handedness) ANOVA identified no significant differences for the first Beta-13 component, but a trend was identified for the second component, $F(1, 69)$ = 3.53, $p$ = .063. Those individuals on death row produced significantly less beta-13 than did individuals in the control group. No significant correlation between Beta-13 and the demographic variables was identified. Figure 2 shows mean Beta-13 magnitude in convicted murderers and controls.

*Beta-16 Activity (16.5-19.45 Hz).* Two components explained 84.85% of the variance in the beta-16 band. The first component loaded heavily in the parietal, occipital, and posterior temporal region (P3, P4, O1, O2, T5, T6). The second component loaded in the frontal, central, and anterior temporal regions (FP1, FP2, F3, F7, F8, C3, C4, T3, T4). Group by handedness ANOVAs found no significant differences in these components, and no correlations were identified between the components and demographic variables. Figure 2 shows mean beta-16 magnitude in convicted murderers and controls.

### Death Row Group 2

*Low-Theta (3.55-5.45 Hz)*. A single component explained 92.17% of the variance in low-theta scores. This component loaded on sites over the entire surface of the scalp. A 2 × 2 (group × handedness) ANOVA revealed that convicted murderers generated less low theta than controls, $F(1, 51) = 42.73, p = .000$. There were no significant correlations between low theta and demographic variables.

*High-Theta (5.5-7.45 Hz)*. A single component explained 94.10% of the variance in high-theta activity. This component was strongly correlated with activity over the entire surface of the scalp. A 2 × 2 (group × handedness) ANOVA revealed a main effect for group, $F(1, 51) = 35.22, p = .000$, such that murderers generated less high-theta. There were no significant correlations between this factor and demographic variables.

*Low-Alpha (7.5-8.45 Hz)*. A single component with strongest loadings in the frontal and central regions (Fp1, Fp2, F3, F4, Cz, C3) explained 93.12% of the variance in low-alpha activity. A 2 × 2 (group × handedness) ANOVA revealed a main effect for group such that murderers had much lower scores on this component than those in the control group, $F(1, 51) = 34.53, p = .000$. There were no significant correlations between the low-alpha component and demographic data.

*Mid-Alpha (8.5-11.45 Hz)*. A single component with loadings in the frontal and central regions (Fz, F3, Cz, C3, C4) explained 92.52% of the variance in mid-alpha activity. A 2 × 2 (group × handedness) ANOVA revealed that murderers generated less mid-alpha compared to controls, $F(1,51) = 39.30, p = .000$. There were no significant correlations between the data and demographic variables.

*High-Alpha (11.5-13.45 Hz)*. A single component with strongest loadings in the frontal and central regions (Fp1, Fp2, Fz, F3, F8, Cz, C3) explained 89.08% of the variance in the high-alpha band. A 2 × 2 (group × handedness) ANOVA showed that controls had much higher scores on this component than did murderers, $F(1, 51) = 27.26, p = .000$.

*Beta-13 (13.5-16.45 Hz).* A single component with loadings in the central and parietal regions (C3, C4, Pz, P4) explained 92.28% of the variance in the Beta-13 band. A 2 × 2 (group × handedness) ANOVA revealed that controls generated more beta-13 compared to murderers, $F(1, 51) = 54.82$, $p = .000$. No significant correlation between beta-13 and the demographic variables was identified.

*Beta-16 (16.5-19.45 Hz).* A single component with loadings in the frontal, central, and parietal regions (Fz, F3, Cz, C3, C4, P3, P4) explained 90.68% of the variance in the Beta-16 band. A 2 × 2 (group × handedness) ANOVA found that murderers produced less Beta-16 than controls, $F(1, 51) = 56.71$, $p = .000$. No correlations were identified between the components and demographic variables.

## Summary of Narrow Band Frequency Analyses

As shown in Table 2, the mean power magnitude of the EEG within each of the frequencies generally was lower for murderers than matched controls. In group 2, these findings were significant across all bands while in group 1, this pattern was significant in high-theta, low- and high-alpha, and in beta-13. For mean power magnitude, generally consistent findings with respect to spatial distribution across both groups were identified in the high-theta, low-alpha, and high-alpha bands.

TABLE 2. Summary of Within-Band Mean Power Magnitude Differences Between Each Group of Murderers and the Control Group

| EEG Frequency | Significant Differences Between Murderers and Controls | | | |
|---|---|---|---|---|
| | Group 1 | | Group 2 | |
| | Direction | Sites | Direction | Sites |
| Low-Theta | n.s. | | M < C*** | Fz, F3, F4, Cz, C4, Pz, P3, P4 |
| High-Theta | M < C* | Fp1, Fp2, Fz, F3, F4, Pz, P3, P4 | M < C*** | Fz, F3, F4, Cz, C4, Pz, P3, P4 |
| Low-Alpha | M < C** | Fp1, Fp2, Fz, F3, F4, Cz, C3, C4 | M < C*** | Fp1, Fp2, F3, F4, Cz, C3 |
| Mid-Alpha | n.s. | | M < C*** | Fz, F3, Cz, C3, C4 |
| High-Alpha | M < C* | FP1, FP2, Fz, F3, F7, F8, C3, C4 | M < C*** | Fp1, Fp2, Fz, F3, F8, Cz, C3 |
| Beta-13 | M < C$^T$ | FP1, FP2, Fz, F3, F7, F8, C3, C4 | M < C*** | C3, C4, Pz, P4 |
| Beta-16 | n.s. | | M < C*** | Fz, F3, Cz, C3, C4, P3, P4 |

* p< .05, ** p < .02, *** p < .001, $^T$ p = .06

## Coherence Analyses

Coherence (i.e., similarity of waveforms) between each set of electrodes was calculated for broad band alpha (7.45-12.45 Hz) using NeuroRep Software (Hudspeth, 1994). Coherences between all possible electrode sites were submitted to a principal components analysis followed by varimax rotation in order to identify patterns of coherences across the groups. This was followed by a t-test to determine which patterns of coherences differentiated murderers and matched controls. Additionally, correlations were run between those patterns of coherences that differentiated between murderers and the comparison group and time spent on death row.

For the first group of murderers, 92.90% of the variance in the pattern of coherence between the murderer group and the comparison group was accounted for by 19 components. Of these, the first 11 components accounted for meaningful proportions of the variance. For the second group of murderers and the comparison group, 94.53% of the variance was explained by 19 components. Of these, the first 12 components accounted for meaningful proportions of the variance. The components which explained meaningful proportions of the variance following varimax rotation were submitted to unpaired t-tests. Of these components, only two were significantly different between murderers and the control group.

A parietal component, the fourth principal component, explained 9.38% of variance in the sample and aligned with coherence between posterior sites. The first group of murderers scored higher on this component ($Mx = .21$, $SDx = .96$) compared to the comparison group ($Mx = -.43$, $SDx = .96$), $t(67) = -1.11$, $p < .01$. This component was nearly identical in structure to the third component between the second group of murderers and the comparison group (11.90% variance explained). The second group of murderers scored higher ($Mx = .32$, $SDx = 1.05$) than the comparison group on this component ($Mx = -.33$, $SDx = .83$), $t(45) = 2.39$, $p < .021$. Figure 3 depicts the structure of coherence across sites in these two components.

A left parietal to frontal component, the eighth principal component, explained 4.64% of the variance. This component aligned with coherence between Pz, P3 and a variety of frontal sites. The first group of murderers scored higher on this component ($Mx = .21$, $SDx = .76$) than the comparison group scored ($Mx = -.43$, $SDx = 1.26$), $t(67) = 2.69$, $p < .009$. This component was nearly identical in structure to the fourth component between the second group of murderers and the comparison

FIGURE 3. Overlap of significant coherence differences in both groups of murderers and the comparison group on sites in the posterior region. These components explained 9.38% of variance between the first group of murderers and the comparison group and 11.90% of the variance between the second group of murderers and the comparison group.

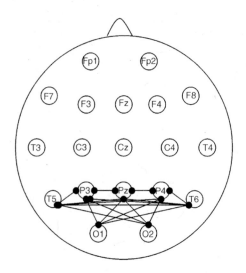

group (8.67% variance explained). The second group of murderers scored higher ($Mx = .31$, $SDx = .94$) than the comparison group scored on this component ($Mx = -.32$, $SDx = .98$), $t(45) = 2.25$, p < .03. Figure 4 depicts the structure of coherence across sites in these two components.

As shown in Figure 4, negative correlations between time spent on death row for a subset of inmates (n = 26) and coherence existed between some frontal and parietal sites (F1-Pz, $r = -.41$, $p = .04$; F7-Pz, $r = -.50$, $p = .01$; F3-Pz, $r = -.42$, $p = .03$; F2-Pz, $r = -.34$, $p = .05$; F7-P3, $r = -.36$, $p = .03$).

## DISCUSSION

This study identified a pattern of suppressed EEG activity in murderers across the entire EEG spectrum in comparison to matched controls. This pattern was particularly marked in anterior regions. Additionally, individuals on death row exhibited increased coherence among certain distal sites and within some posterior regions as compared to controls.

FIGURE 4. Overlap of significant differences in both groups of murderers and the comparison group on the principal component loading on regions between left parietal sites and frontal sites. These components explained 4.64% of the variance between the first group of murderers and the comparison group and 8.67% of the variance between the second group of murderers and the comparison groups. Dotted lines indicate significant negative correlations between time spent on death row for a subset of inmates (n=26) and coherence (F1-Pz, r = −.41, p = .04; F7-Pz, r = −.50, p = .01; F3-Pz, r = −.42, p = .03; F2-Pz, r = −.34, p = .05; F7-P3, r = −.36, p = .03).

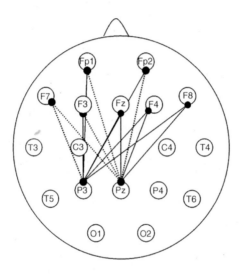

Both groups of murderers exhibited less high theta than matched controls in frontal (Fz, F3, F4) and parietal (Pz, P3, P4) regions. As time served on death row is reportedly correlated with cognitive impairment, this finding was hypothesized. This effect was localized primarily to frontal regions, suggesting that this high-theta may be frontal midline theta. A suppression of frontal midline theta would support inmates' self-reported decline in cognitive abilities and attention, and perhaps particularly their self-reported memory impairment.

Both murderer groups exhibited less low alpha than the matched control group in frontal (Fp1, Fp2, F3, F4) and central (Cz, C4) regions; this countered what was expected. It was hypothesized that these individuals would generate more low alpha compared to controls, as inmates have been found to report drowsiness, listlessness, and mental slowness. If there was suppression of low alpha, it may be a carryover from the high-theta band or may be in reaction to generalized arousal. It also may be related to the overall suppression of EEG that has been reported in studies of mental decline with aging (Edman, Brunovsky, Sjögren, Wallin, & Matousek, 2003).

We expected that individuals on death row would have less high alpha as compared to controls, as they often have cognitive impairments which we speculated are most likely associated with changes in their ability to maintain attention. In both groups of murderers, mean magnitude of high alpha was suppressed in the frontal lobes as compared to controls. We hypothesized that both beta-13 and beta-16 would be suppressed in murderers as compared to matched controls. In beta-13 at C3, C4 there was a trend towards this pattern in group 1, and in group 2 this trend reached significance. The suppression of beta-16 was only significant in Group 2.

The finding of suppression of waveforms, particularly in the frontal regions, supports findings in PET research (Raine et al., 1997; Raine et al., 1998). As frontal regions are often damaged in closed head injuries (Richardson, 1990), it was not surprising to find abnormal EEG patterns in these individuals. However, since these groups were compared to a matched control group with neurological impairments, the presence of injury would not explain this overall difference.

The frontal lobes are involved in behavioral inhibition, judgment, self-monitoring, advance planning, and cognitive flexibility (Kolb & Wishaw, 1995). This suggests that frontal lobe differences in the murderers may have put these individuals at risk for engaging in violent, unlawful behaviors. This risk may be increased with a comorbidity of child abuse, serious mental illness, or substance abuse (Nestor, 1992). One or more of these factors is commonly found in the histories of convicted murderers (Raine et al., 1994; Raine et al., 1998).

The overall suppression of EEG waveforms in the murderers, which was significant in all bands in Group 2 and significant in most bands of EEG in Group 1, is similar to studies of elderly patients with brain abnormalities (Salokangas, Loikkanen, & Santala, 1990). Given the stressful experience of living on death rows and the research suggesting that extreme stress increases cognitive aging (Shanan & Shahar, 1983), this finding was not unexpected. To pursue this issue further, correlations were calculated between the EEG variables involved in this study and the actual time on death row. The latter information was available for a subset of 26 individuals from the murderers. There were only two significant correlations. Time spent on death row was correlated with more low theta in posterior regions. However, time spent on death row was not correlated significantly with EEG in any other band. This may be due to the small size of the group for whom time spent on death row was available. The positive correlation between low theta magnitude in the posterior regions and time spent on death row may provide support for Shanan and Shahar's argument regarding stress and cognitive aging.

We expected that coherence would be greater in murderers than matched controls, and we found this pattern in both groups. Evans and Park (1997) identified a pattern of abnormally increased coherence in their study of murderers on death rows, and suggested that the increase indicated decreased cortical differentiation as is commonly observed in individuals with a history of brain injury. However, as both groups of murderers in this study showed increased coherence with respect to the neurologically impaired control group it is possible that the observed effect is not due to brain injury alone.

Based on Evans and Park (1997), we hypothesized that individuals on death row would have more impairment between distal cortical regions than matched controls would have. As shown in Figure 4, there was clear evidence of a difference in coherence between distal regions in neurologically impaired controls and murderers in both groups. Between left and central parietal and frontal regions murderers exhibited substantially higher coherence than controls exhibited. However, there was a negative correlation between time spent on death row and coherence between the parietal site and frontal sites such that the longer individuals spent on death row the lower their coherence in these regions. These findings suggest that not all of the differences between the murderers and comparison group can be attributed to time spent on death row.

Unexpectedly, murderers exhibited greater posterior intrahemispheric coherence among several sites compared to matched controls. This finding has been associated in the literature with a decrease in alertness in individuals with brain abnormalities (Edman et al., 2003), and may be related to inmates' reports of listlessness and decreases in alertness.

We expected murderers would have more right than left hemisphere abnormalities of coherence. We did not replicate this finding from Evans and Park (1997). However, that study compared murderers with brain damage to a normative database. In the current study we attempted to contrast murderers with matched neurologically impaired controls. In this study, the principal components analysis revealed a pattern of coherence across all groups between the right temporal regions and frontal regions (see Figure 5, right temporal and anterior sites) which may be the pattern of coherence identified in the study by Evans

FIGURE 5. Overlapping regions of coherence that did not distinguish between two groups of murderers and the matched control group ranked by percent of variance explained.

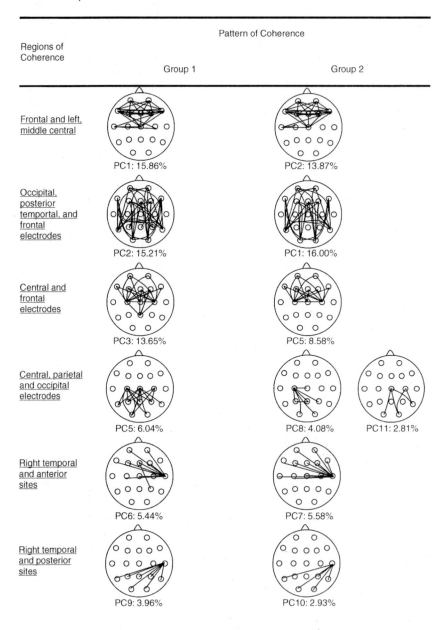

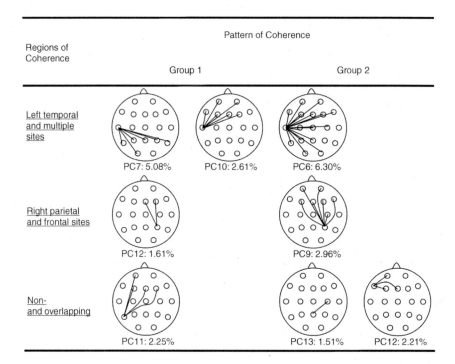

Pattern of Coherence

Regions of Coherence

Group 1 — Group 2

Left temporal and multiple sites — PC7: 5.08% — PC10: 2.61% — PC6: 6.30%

Right parietal and frontal sites — PC12: 1.61% — PC9: 2.96%

Non- and overlapping — PC11: 2.25% — PC13: 1.51% — PC12: 2.21%

and Park (1997). In the earlier study, they may have identified a pattern of coherence that generally is associated with brain injury rather than more specifically with violent behavior.

This study had several limitations. The majority of inmates were selected for QEEG assessment due to independent evidence of factors in their background which put them at risk for brain damage, so care must be taken when generalizing to the death row population at large. Overall, the power spectrum in Group 2 was significantly smaller than either the control group or Group 1. Statistical testing did not identify any outliers, but it is possible that one or more anomalous cases swayed the final results. Additionally, the subset of individuals for whom time spent on death row was available was quite small ($n = 26$); a replication of this study with a larger sample size would be valuable.

Although the use of the neurologically impaired matched controls with no history of violent behavior has been suggested by several studies, it would be useful to conduct a study comparing murderers to both an average population and to matched neurologically impaired controls. A study in which murderers are compared to matched neurologically impaired controls with a history of substance abuse or abuse as children, but no history of violence would also add to this literature.

In conclusion, this study identified a pattern of suppressed EEG activity in murderers in comparison to matched controls. This pattern was particularly marked in anterior regions. Additionally, individuals on death row revealed a pattern of increased coherence among distal sites and within the posterior regions. In combination, these results suggest that murderers experience less cortical differentiation and lower levels of alertness than neurological impaired matched controls experience. Additionally, there were certain other changes in their EEG spectrum and coherences that support murderers' frequently self-reported symptoms of cognitive and physical decline. Some of the group differences were unrelated to time spent on death row. This suggests that the changes in their EEGs can be attributed to factors that occurred before they spent time on death row, as well as factors associated with spending time on death row. Any future study of EEG should address this important issue. Although it may be impossible to completely tease apart the contributions of history, brain injury, and experience on death row, there is evidence that each of these factors contributes to the overall pattern of QEEG findings in these individuals.

## REFERENCES

Adler, G., Bramesfeld, A., & Jajcevic, A. (1999). Mild cognitive impairment in old-age depression is associated with increased EEG slow-wave power. *Neuropsychobiology, 40*, 219-222.

Arrigo, B. A., & Fowler, C. R. (2001). The "death row community": A community psychology perspective. *Deviant Behavior: An Interdisciplinary Journal, 22*, 43-71.

Barceló, F., & Gale, A. (1997). Electrophysiological measures of cognition in biological psychiatry: Some cautionary notes. *International Journal of Neuroscience, 92*, 219-240.

Barceló, F., Gale, A., & Hall, M. (1995). Multichannel EEG power reflects information processing and attentional demands during visual orienting. *Journal of Psychophysiology, 9*, 32-44.

Blueston, H., & McGahee, C. L. (1962). Reaction to extreme stress: Impending death by execution. *American Journal of Psychiatry, 119*, 393-396.

Bonczar, T. P., & Snell, T. L. (2003). *Capital punishment, 2002*. Bureau of Justice Statistics Bulletin (Bureau of Justice Statistics Publication No. NCJ 201848). Washington, DC.

Crawford, H. J., Clarke, S. W., & Kitner-Triolo, M. (1996). Self-generated happy and sad emotions in low and highly hypnotizable persons during waking and hypnosis: Laterality and regional EEG activity differences. *International Journal of Psychophysiology, 24,* 239-266.

Crawford, H. J., Knebel, T. F., Vendemia, J. M. C., Kaplan, L., & Ratcliff, B. (1995). EEG activation patterns during tracking and decision-making tasks: Differences between low and high sustained adults. *Proceedings of the 8th International Symposium on Aviation Psychology* (pp. 886-890). Columbus, OH.

Cunningham, M. D., & Vigen, M. P. (2002). Death row inmate characteristics, adjustment, and confinement: A critical review of the literature. *Behavioral Sciences and the Law, 20,* 191-210.

Duffy, F., H., Bartels, P. H., & Neff, R. (1986). A response to Oken and Chiappa. *Neuroscience Issues, 19,* 494-497.

Edman, A., Brunovsky, M., Sjögren, M., Wallin, A., & Matousek, M. (2003). Objective measurement of alertness level in dementia. *Dementia & Geriatric Cognitive Disorders, 15,* 212-217.

Evans, J. R., & Park, N. (1997). Quantitative EEG findings among men convicted of murder. *Journal of Neurotherapy, 2* (2), 31-39.

Freedman, D., & Hemenway, D. (2000). Precursors of lethal violence: A death row sample. *Social Science and Medicine, 50,* 1757-1770.

Frierson, R. L., Schwartz-Watts, D. M., Morgan, D. W., & Malone, T. D. (1998). Capital versus noncapital murderers. *Journal of the American Academy of Psychiatry and Law, 26,* 403-410.

Gallermore, J. L., & Pantón, M. A. (1972). Inmate responses to lengthy death row confinement. *American Journal of Psychiatry, 129,* 167-172.

Hermann, W. M., & Schaerer, E. (1986). Pharmaco-EEG: Computer EEG analysis to describe the projection of drug effects on a functional cerebral level in humans. In F. H. Lopes da Silva, W. Strom van Leeuwen, & A. Remond (Eds.), *Handbook of electroencephalography and clinical neurophysiology* (pp. 385-445). Amsterdam: Elsevier.

Hudspeth, W. J. (1994). Neuroelectric eigenstructures of mental representation. In D. S. Levine, & M. Aparicio (Eds.), *Neural networks for knowledge representation and inference* (pp. 419-446). Hillsdale, NJ: Lawrence Erlbaum Associates.

Inouye, T., Ishihara, T., Shinosaki, K., Toi, S., & Ukai, S. (1988). EEG characteristics of frontal midline theta activity. In D. Giannitrapani & L. Murri (Eds.), *The EEG of mental activities* (pp. 136-148). Basel, Switzerland: S. Karger.

Ishihara, T., & Yoshi, N. (1972). Multivariate analytic study of EEG and mental activity in juvenile delinquents. *Electroencephalography and Clinical Neurophysiology, 33,* 71-80.

Jasper, H. H. (1958). The ten-twenty electrode system of the International Federation. *Electroencephalography and Clinical Neurophysiology, 10,* 371-375.

Jastak, S., & Wilkinson, G. (1984). *Wide Range Achievement Test-Revised.* Wilmington, DE: Jastak Associates, Inc.

Johnson, R. (1979). Under the sentence of death: The psychology of death row confinement. *Law & Psychology Review, 5,* 141-192.

Klimesch, W. (1996). Memory processes, brain oscillations and EEG synchronization. *International Journal of Psychophysiology, 24,* 61-100.

Kolb, B., & Wishaw, I. (1995). *Fundamentals of human neuropsychology.* New York: W. Freeman & Company.

Ladds, B., & Trachtenberg, D. (1995). Letter to the editor: Glucose metabolism in murderers. *Biological Psychiatry, 38,* 341.

Lewis, D. O., Pincus, J. H., Bard, B., Richardson, E., Prichep, L. S., Feldman, M., et al. (1988). Neuropsychiatric, psychoeducational, and family characteristics of 14 juveniles condemned to death in the United States. *American Journal of Psychiatry, 145,* 584-589.

Lewis, D., Pincus, J., Feldman, M., Jackson, L., & Bard, B. (1986). Psychiatric, neurological, and psychoeducational characteristics of 15 death row inmates in the United States. *American Journal of Psychiatry, 143,* 838-845.

Mann, C. A., Sterman, M. B., & Kaiser, D. A. (1996). Suppression of EEG rhythmic frequencies during somato-motor and visuo-motor behavior. *International Journal of Psychophysiology, 23* (1-2), 1-7.

Mecklinger, A., Kramer, A. F., & Strayer, D. L. (1992). Event related potentials and EEG components in a semantic memory search task. *Psychophysiology, 29,* 104-119.

Mizuki, Y., Kajimura, N., Kai, S., & Suetsugi, M. (1992). Differential responses to mental stress in high and low anxious normal humans assessed by frontal midline theta activity. *International Journal of Psychophysiology, 12,* 169-178.

Nestor, P. G. (1992). Neuropsychological and clinical correlates of murder and other forms of extreme violence in forensic psychiatric populations. *The Journal of Nervous and Mental Disease, 180,* 218-223.

Raine, A., Buchsbaum, M., & LaCasse, L. (1997). Brain abnormalities in murderers indicated by Positron Emission Tomorgraphy. *Biological Psychiatry, 42,* 495-508.

Raine, A., Buchsbaum, M. S., Stanley, J., Lottenberg, S., Abel, L., & Stoddard, J. (1994). Selective reductions in prefrontal glucose metabolism in murderers. *Biological Psychiatry, 36,* 365-373.

Raine, A, Meloy, J. R., Bihrle, A., Stoddard, J., LaCasse, L., & Buchsbaum, M. S. (1998). Reduced prefrontal and increased subcortical brain functioning assessed using positron emission tomography in predatory and affective murderers. *Behavioral Sciences and the Law, 16,* 319-332.

Ramos, J., Corsi-Cabrera, M., Guevara, M. A., & Arce, G. (1993). EEG activity during cognitive activity in women. *International Journal of Neuroscience, 69,* 185-195.

Richardson, J. T. (1990). *Clinical and neuropsychological aspects of closed head injury.* Bristol, PA: Taylor & Francis, Inc.

Salokangas, R., Loikkanen, T, & Santala, H. (1990). The patients of special psychogeriatric ward: Psychosocial situation, clinical disorder and results of treatment. *Psychiatria, Fennica, 21,* 175-188.

Schacter, D. L. (1977). EEG theta waves and psychological phenomena: A review and analysis. *Biological Psychology, 5,* 47-82.

Shanan, J., & Shahar, O. (1983). Cognitive and personality functioning of Jewish Holocaust survivors during the midlife transition (46-65) in Israel. *Archiv Für Psychologie, 135,* 275-294.

Soininen, H., Partanen, J., Laulumaa, V., Paakkonen, A., Helkala, E. L., & Riekkinen, P. J. (1991). Serial EEG in Alzheimer's disease: 3-year follow-up and clinical outcome. *Electroencephalography Clinics in Neurophysiology, 79,* 342-348.

Sterman, M. B., Mann, C. A., Kaiser, D. A., & Suyenobu, B. Y. (1994). Multiband topographic EEG analysis of a simulated visuomotor aviation task. *International Journal of Psychophysiology, 16* (1), 49-56.

Thatcher, R., Walker, R., & Guidice, S. (1987). Human cerebral hemispheres develop at different rates and ages. *Science, 236*, 1110-1113.

Tucker, D. M., & Roth, D. L. (1984). Factoring the coherence matrix: Patterning of the frequency-specific covariance in a multichannel EEG. *Psychophysiology, 21*, 228-236.

U.S. Department of Justice (2004). *Capital punishment in the United States, 1973-2002* [Data file]. Ann Arbor, MI: Inter-university Consortium for Political and Social Research [producer and distributor].

Wilkinson, G. (1993). *Wide Range Achievement Test 3*. Wilmington, DE: Wide Range, Inc.

Williamson, P. C., Merskey, H., Morrison, S., Rabeheru, K., Fox, H., Wands, K., et al. (1990). Quantitative electro-encephalographic correlates of cognitive decline in normal elderly subjects. *Archives of Neurology, 47*, 1185-1188.

# The qEEG in the Lie Detection Problem: The Localization of Guilt?

## Kirtley E. Thornton, PhD

**SUMMARY.** Previous attempts by the author to discern if the qEEG could be an effective instrument in the detection of a lie resulted in positive results (100% effective, 73% of the time; Thornton, 1995). The procedure failed to make a decision in 4 of the 15 events being examined. A new design was created which requires no verbal response of the participant. The participant in the present study was presented with four instructions: (a) allow yourself to be anxious, (b) listen to stories of events of which you have no direct experience or knowledge, (c) listen to stories of self-reported true (real crimes) events which you participated in and feel guilty about your participation, and (d) block the real crime stories (events provided by participant) as they are read to you. The participant's eyes were closed during the entire collection of data and no verbal response was elicited. Analysis of the different cognitive/emotional states with qEEG measures revealed an intriguing predominant pattern of left hemisphere/posterior (dorsal) activation for the experience of anxiety, right hemisphere (right temporal, in particular) activation for the experiencing of guilt and more centrally located activations when the participant attempted to block the real stories. *[Article copies available for a fee from The Haworth Document Delivery Service: 1-800-HAWORTH. E-mail address: <docdelivery@haworthpress.com> Website: <http://www.HaworthPress.com> © 2005 by The Haworth Press, Inc. All rights reserved.]*

Kirtley E. Thornton is affiliated with The Center for Health Psychology, a mental health clinic in Plainfield, New Jersey.

Address correspondence to: Kirtley E. Thornton, Suite 2A, 2509 Park Avenue, South Plainfield, NJ 07080 (E-mail: ket@chp-neurotherapy.com).

[Haworth co-indexing entry note]: "The qEEG in the Lie Detection Problem: The Localization of Guilt?" Thornton, Kirtley E. Co-published simultaneously in *Journal of Neurotherapy* (The Haworth Medical Press, an imprint of The Haworth Press, Inc.) Vol. 9, No. 3, 2005, pp. 31-43; and: *Forensic Applications of QEEG and Neurotherapy* (ed: James R. Evans) The Haworth Medical Press, an imprint of The Haworth Press, Inc., 2005, pp. 31-43. Single or multiple copies of this article are available for a fee from The Haworth Document Delivery Service [1-800-HAWORTH, 9:00 a.m. - 5:00 p.m. (EST). E-mail address: docdelivery@haworthpress.com].

Available online at http://www.haworthpress.com/web/JN
© 2005 by The Haworth Press, Inc. All rights reserved.
doi:10.1300/J184v09n03_03

**KEYWORDS.** qEEG, lie detection, guilt, innocence

## INTRODUCTION

The history of lie detection by psychophysiological methods has been fraught with problems of human judgment, reliability and validity. Early Hindu medical records (900 B.C.) noted the use of blushing (facial vasodilation) in the detection of guilt (Ben-Shakhar & Furedy, 1990). A most impressive case is attributed to Eristratus, a physician to Alexander the Great, who determined by use of the tumultuous rhythm of the heart that the crown prince of the Seleucid court in Syria was guilty of a sexual relationship with his stepmother. Months later a child was born (Trovillo, 1939, p. 850), confirming for the first time the use of physiological measures in the detection of deception.

William Marston (1917) was the first proponent of lie detection machines. In the Frye versus United States, 54 App. D. C. 46, 47, 293 F. 1013, 1014 case (1923) the rule was established that expert opinion based on a scientific technique is inadmissible unless the technique is "generally accepted" as reliable in the relevant scientific community. Marston's introduction of blood pressure to assess lie detection was accepted by the court as "generally accepted" in this landmark legal case establishing the Frye standard. The polygraph was used and promoted by the Berkeley, California police department in the 1930s. Dozens of polygraph schools sprang up around the country. The industry thrived, with three branches: pre-employment testing, criminal investigation and counterintelligence.

The main methodologies of lie detection are the Control Question Technique (CQT) and the Guilty Knowledge Test (GKT). Descriptions of the following methodologies can be found in the NASA report (Fienberg, 2002) and a publication by Ben-Shakhar and Furedy (1990). The CQT methodology involves construction of a control question which has greater emotional impact than the crime-relevant question (assuming the participant is innocent). Thus the participant may be asked "Did you ever do anything you were ashamed of"? The questions are constructed to be vague and intended to elicit an anxious response. If the reaction to the control question is greater than the relevant question (relevant to the crime), the participant is deemed to be telling the truth. If the reaction to the relevant question is greater than the control question, it is concluded that the participant is lying.

A variant of the CQT methodology (the Directed Lie Test, DLT) asks the participant to lie to a control question (e.g., "Have you ever broken a rule"?) and simultaneously to think about the time they did break a rule. If the participant's reactions to relevant (to the crime) questions are judged by officials to be larger than their reactions to directed-lie questions, the participant is deemed to be lying.

The GKT involves direct questions which are posed to the participant. These questions involve information that only the guilty participant would know. For example, the participant is asked "Was she wearing a black dress that night"? Multiple choice items are generally presented and the participant's response is compared on the "concealed information" (that which the guilty participant would be aware of) to the neutral items. If the participant shows greater physiological response to the "concealed items," guilt is presumed.

The NASA review (Fienberg, 2002) represents the most thorough review of the literature in this area. The report described many different problems in the area.

> For example, in different studies, when a cutoff is used that yields a false positive rate of roughly 10 percent, the sensitivity–the proportion of guilty examinees correctly identified–ranges from 43 to 100 percent. This range is only moderately narrower, roughly 64 to 100 percent, in studies reporting a cutoff that resulted in 30 percent of truthful examinees being judged deceptive. (Fienberg, 2002, p. 105)

> In screening populations with very low base rates of deceptive individuals, even an extremely high percentage of correct classifications can give very unsatisfactory results. This point is illustrated in Table 2-1 (in Chapter 2), which presents an example of a test with an accuracy index of 0.90 that makes 99.5 percent correct classifications in a hypothetical security screening situation, yet lets 8 of 10 spies pass the screen. (Fienberg, 2002, p. 126)

The NASA report concluded:

> Thus, the range of accuracy indexes, from 0.81 to 0.91, that covers the bulk of polygraph research studies, is in our judgment an overestimate of likely accuracy in field application, even when highly trained examiners and reasonably well standardized testing procedures are used. It is impossible, however, to quantify how much of

an overestimate these numbers represent because of limitations in the data. In our judgment, however, reliance on polygraph testing to perform in practical applications at a level at or above Accuracy Index = 0.90 is not warranted on the basis of either scientific theory or empirical data. Many committee members would place this upper bound considerably lower. (Fienberg, 2002, p. 126)

## Popular Lie Detectors

The movement into the popular arena for lie detectors has seen the advent of voice recognition software which presumably will tell if a person is lying. Internet ads for lie detection devices are now common and a device from Israel purports to tell you if your spouse really loves you while he or she talks to you, even providing a rating scale for love. Many of the commercial lie detection devices are, by and large, sensitive to issues of anxiety and tension. Research conducted by the Department of Defense (Cestaro, 1996; Cestaro & Dollins, 1994; Janniro & Cestaro, 1996) has concluded that voice analysis lie detection software does not provide hit rates above chance levels. NASA's report (Fienberg, 2002) underscores the lack of validity of this particular method.

Traditional lie detection methodologies have relied upon autonomic and somatic nervous system response: cardiovascular (i.e., changes in heart rate and blood pressure), electrodermal (i.e., changes in the electrical properties of the skin that vary with the activity of the eccrine sweat gland), and respiratory. Modern electrophysiological measurements (event-related potentials–P300; Rosenfeld, Angell, Johnson, & Qian, 1991) have also been applied to the problem, with similar hit rates to traditional approaches (MacLaren, 2001).

These traditional approaches have several limitations: (a) the time delay between the experiencing of lying and the physiological response, (b) the number of physiological variables being collected, (c) the requirement of a verbal response, and/or (d) the variables can be under the control of the participant. The author designed an approach which employs the qEEG (which does not have the time delay problem), increases the number of available physiological variables, does not require a verbal response and is too difficult for the participant to control (as there are about 3,000 variables being measured). The goal would be a "foolproof" lie detector test which never asks the participant to answer a question.

In this approach, a variance of the GKT technique, a participant is read true stories concerning an event where guilt is reported and stories of events or crimes about which they have no knowledge. This approach differs from the GKT technique through the collection of qEEG data and the lack of verbal response by the participant. An additional advantage of this design is that story reading involves more time than that required to answer a question, allowing for extensive data collection.

This method also controls for anxiety and blocking, two problems that have plagued traditional methods. The participant provides an anxiety control condition, producing this emotion on his or her own for a minute or two, and a faking or blocking control condition in which a participant is asked to "block" in whatever manner possible the hearing or impact of a story about a real, self-reported, guilt-provoking event in his or her life. Blocking may involve a lack of cognitive processing of verbal information or a suppression of normal emotional responses to a story. How well a participant was able to block a story was not measured for this study.

## METHOD

### Participant

The participant was a 23-year-old Caucasian female who volunteered for the project. She was not reimbursed for her participation. There was no history of brain injury, neurological disease or other medical history which could affect her qEEG.

### Apparatus

The qEEG was acquired using the NRS-24 recording equipment (Lexicor Medical Technology, Inc.) and a 10-20 system Electro-cap with a linked-ears reference. Sampling rate was 256 samples per second, which allows for examination of up to the 64 Hz range with a 60 Hz notch filter. Software filters provided high and low frequency passes at 0.5 and 64 Hz (3dB points), respectively. Signals were subjected to a Fast Fourier Transform (FFT) using cosine-tapered windows which output spectral magnitude in peak-to-peak microvolts as a function of frequency. The bandwidths analyzed were Delta: 0-4 Hz, Theta: 4-8 Hz, Alpha: 8-13 Hz, Beta1: 13-32 Hz, Beta2: 32-64 Hz. Scalp locations were prepped with rubbing alcohol and Nu-Prep and all site impedances were below 5 K ohms, and within 1.5 K of each other. Gain was set to 32,000 and epoch length was set to 1 second. Data were visually analyzed for artifact and epochs marked for deletion when artifact was evident.

### Activation Measures

The following spectral indices were calculated for each recording condition:

1. Average absolute magnitude in microvolts in a band.
2. Average relative magnitude in a band at a site, calculated by dividing absolute magnitude of a particular band by total microvolts in all bands.
3. Peak Amplitude: Peak amplitude in microvolts in a band.
4. Peak Frequency: Peak frequency of a band.

Symmetry: Peak amplitude symmetry between homotopic sites in a band [i.e., defined as $(A - B)/(A + B)$].

### Connectivity Measures

Coherence is the average similarity between the waveforms (of a particular band) from two locations over a one-second period of time conceptualized as the strength/number of connections between two locations.

Phase is the time lag between two waveforms from two locations (of a particular band), defined by how soon after the beginning of an epoch a particular waveform from location 1 is matched by that from location 2.

### Procedure

The participant was asked to provide five stories concerning her life about which she felt guilty. These were considered to be real crimes.

The real crimes that the participant committed involved knocking a friend's TV off a refrigerator and not taking responsibility for it, lying to a friend about what she was planning to do on New Year's Eve (and thus avoided being with the friend), lying to a potential date about being grounded because she didn't want to go on a date with him, lying to her mother about drinking, and an additional story the participant did not want revealed. The author constructed five additional stories which had no relevance to the participant's life. For example, the stories involved a breaking and entering crime, murder of a spouse following a suspected affair, a covered up death following a hit and run, stealing money at a New Year's Eve party with friends and shoplifting during Christmas.

EEG data were gathered continuously, first during an eyes-closed, resting condition, then while the participant was asked to experience anxiety, and then while listening to stories orally presented by the examiner (lasting 45 to 120 seconds). The reading of the stories alternated between reading the five false crimes and then the five true crimes (i.e., false crime, true crime, false crime, etc.). This allowed for analysis of changes across repetitions. However, in this study, only the first exposure to the stories was subsequently employed in the analysis. The possible habituation of response pattern was not examined. The participant's eyes were closed in all conditions and instructions were: relax, with your eyes closed (condition one), allow yourself to be anxious (condition two), listen (conditions three and four), and block the stories (condition five).

## Statistical Procedures

For the four comparisons the means and standard deviations (SD) of the (a) condition (test condition) were obtained. The mean of the (b) condition (control condition) then was compared to the (a) condition, employing the SD of the (a) condition. For example, the mean and SD of the (a) condition were employed to calculate the Z score increase of the variable when the participant experienced anxiety (b) condition. The figures present the standard deviation differences for the variables. The criteria for significance were a greater than one SD increase from the (a) to the (b) conditions.

## RESULTS

Listening to a real crime was compared to listening to a false crime, blocking while a real crime is read, and the anxiety condition. The anxiety condition was also compared to an eyes closed rest baseline. Spectral means were compared by using the standard deviation of the control condition. The control condition is listed first in each figure. Darkened circles in each figure represent preferential activation at this location from control to test condition. It is of some interest to note that the coherence and phase measures did not provide any significant results.

### Eyes-Closed Resting Condition vs. Anxious Condition

Figure 1 presents the comparison between the eyes-closed resting condition and the anxious condition. This comparison indicated all significant activations were in the higher Beta frequency range (32-64 Hz) especially in posterior regions (nine total activations at O1, O2 and T6 in particular). In addition, consistent (across different measures) activations were noted in the T3-T5 section and T4. There were 13 significant variables in the left hemisphere and seven in the right hemisphere. The participant provided an intensity rating of 8 (out of 10) for the anxious feeling. Only the participant's statement was relied upon for this experience.

FIGURE 1. Eyes-Closed Resting Condition vs. Anxious Condition

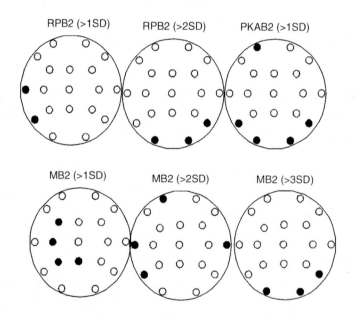

**Blackened Circles indicate that the location was different from the comparison condition by the amount specified above the individual head figure.**
**RPB2: Relative Power Beta2  PKAB2: Peak Amplitude Beta2  MB2: Magnitude Beta2**
**Beta1: 13-32 Hz  Beta2: 32-64 Hz**
>1SD: greater than 1 Standard Deviation
>2SD: greater than 2 Standard Deviations
>3SD: greater than 3 Standard Deviations

## *Hearing False Crimes vs. Real Crimes*

Figure 2 presents the comparison between the hearing false crimes and hearing real crimes condition. This comparison points to a frontal/temporal activation pattern in the higher frequency (32-64 Hz) occurring along the F7-T3-T5 and F8-T4-T6 paths. The strongest (in terms of standard deviations) activation was the T4 location with the peak amplitude of Beta2 providing a greater than two standard deviations difference and the magnitude Beta2 measure showing a greater than four standard deviation difference from the hearing false crimes condition. There were five significant activations in the left hemisphere and seven in the right hemisphere.

FIGURE 2. Hearing False Crimes vs. Hearing Real Crimes

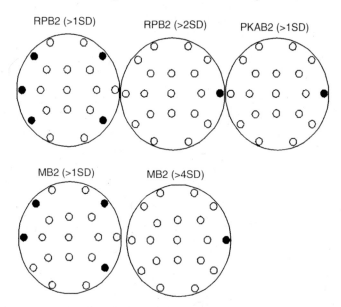

RPB2 (>1SD)    RPB2 (>2SD)    PKAB2 (>1SD)

MB2 (>1SD)    MB2 (>4SD)

**Blackened Circles indicate that the location was different from the comparison condition by the amount specified above the individual head figure.**
**RPB2: Relative Power Beta2    PKAB2: Peak Amplitude Beta2**
**MB2: Magnitude Beta2**
>1SD: greater than 1 Standard Deviation
>2SD: greater than 2 Standard Deviations
>4SD: greater than 4 Standard Deviations

## Hearing a Real Crime vs. Trying to Block While Hearing a Real Crime

Figure 3 presents the comparison between the hearing a real crime and trying to block the examiner's message while hearing a real crime. When the participant tried to block the real crime story, the pattern of response was a much more centrally located activation pattern and minimal activation of the T4 location. The participant reported that she was trying to block the incoming information by distracting herself with other thoughts. Furthermore, the response pattern was bilateral (20 in the left hemisphere and 22 in the right hemisphere), and was more centrally located (30 in central locations and 24 in more laterally located positions). Whereas in the first two comparisons all the significant results were focused on the Beta2 bandwidth, this comparison resulted in a preponderance of differences in the Beta1 bandwidth.

FIGURE 3. Hearing a Real Crime vs. Trying to Block When Hearing a Real Crime

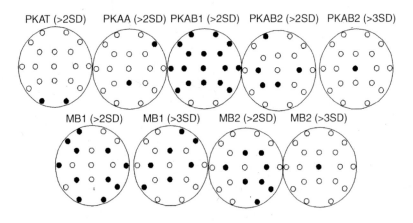

Blackened Circles indicate that the location was different from the comparison condition by the amount specified above the individual head figure.
PKAT: Peak amplitude Theta PKAA: Peak Amplitude Alpha
PKAB1: Peak Amplitude Beta1 PKAB2: Peak Amplitude Beta2
MB1: Magnitude Beta1 MB2: Magnitude Beta2
Beta1: 13-32 Hz Beta2: 32-64 Hz
>2SD: greater than 2 Standard Deviations
>3SD: greater than 3 Standard Deviations

## Anxiety Condition vs. Hearing a Real Crime

Figure 4 presents the comparison between the anxiety condition and hearing a real crime. In this comparison, the participant's response to the real crime was more focused on the T4 and C4 locations. The right hemisphere pattern was considerably more prevalent as there were only two activations in the left hemisphere and nine in the right hemisphere. All of the significant findings involved symmetry measures (both Beta1 and Beta2 bandwidths).

## DISCUSSION

This participant presented a unique set of responses to the different cognitive/emotional tasks. Generally, all the tasks elicited activity in the higher Beta frequency range (32-64 Hz). The author's experience in artifacting was relied upon to discern EMG artifact and delete the affected epochs from analysis. However, EMG artifact could be considered a relevant source of information in the lie detection situation, as it could indicate tension reflected in the muscle system. A participant may characteristically tighten muscles in the neck when they lie, the so-called "tell" involved in poker games.

Temporal lobe activity appeared to be an especially significant issue in this case. The experience of anxiety raised posterior Beta2 activity in

FIGURE 4. Anxiety Condition vs. Hearing Real Crimes

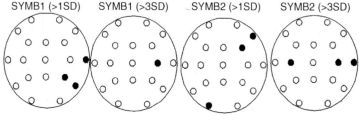

SYMB1 (>1SD)    SYMB1 (>3SD)    SYMB2 (>1SD)    SYMB2 (>3SD)

Blackened Circles indicate that the location was different from the comparison
condition by the amount specified above the individual head figure.
SYMB1: Symmetry Beta1 SYMB2: Symmetry Beta2
Beta1: 13-32 Hz Beta2: 32-64 Hz
>1SD: greater than 1 Standard Deviation
>3SD: greater than 3 Standard Deviations

more left hemisphere/posterior locations along the occipital-temporal locations. Temporal activations were confined to the left temporal location (T3) and there was a left hemisphere focus to the activations. As the participant listened to real crimes (vs. false crimes) the focus of the activations shifted to the right temporal location (T4). The focus of the activations was in the right hemisphere, a pattern different from the anxiety condition. From this line of reasoning, guilt may be seen as a right hemisphere (in particular, right temporal) activation pattern and anxiety as a left hemisphere/posterior pattern. Figure 3 (anxiety vs. real crime) further supports the concept that guilt has a right hemisphere manifestation (all symmetry measures).

When the participant attempted to block the inflow of the message (Figure 3), she activated the central locations apparently by creating internal thought patterns. The separation of anxiety from guilt is clear in Figure 4 and strongly points to a right hemisphere–and in particular a right temporal involvement in the experience of guilt. In this participant, the qEEG approach to the lie detection problem has provided encouraging results for further research and development.

## REFERENCES

Ben-Shakur, G., & Furedy, J. J. (1990). *Theories and applications in the detection of deception.* New York: Springer-Verlag.

Cestaro, V. L. (1996). *A comparison of accuracy rates between detection of deception examinations using the polygraph and the computer voice stress analyzer in a mock crime scenario.* (Report No. DoDPI95-R-0004). Washington, DC: Department of Defense Polygraph Institute.

Cestaro, V. L., & Dollins, A. B. (1994). *An analysis of voice responses for the detection of deception.* (Report No. DoDPI94-R-0001). Washington, DC: Department of Defense Polygraph Institute.

Fienberg, S. (Chair). (2002). *The polygraph and lie detection.* Committee to review the scientific evidence on the polygraph, NASA Report, 2002. Washington, DC: The National Academies Press.

Janniro, M. J., & Cestaro, V. L. (1996). *Effectiveness of detection of deception examinations using the computer voice stress analyzer* (Report No. DODPI96-R-0005). Washington, DC: Department of Defense Polygraph Institute.

MacLaren, V. V. (2001). A quantitative review of the guilty knowledge test. *Journal of Applied Psychology, 86,* 674-683.

Marston, W. M. (1917). Systolic blood pressure changes in deception. *Journal of Experimental Psychology, 2,* 143-163.

Rosenfeld, J. P., Angell, A., Johnson, M., & Qian, J. H. (1991). An ERP-based, control-question lie detector analog: Algorithms for discriminating effects within individuals' average waveforms. *Psychophysiology, 28,* 319-335.

Thornton, K. (1995). The anatomy of the lie: A QEEG investigation into lie detection. *Journal of Offender Rehabilitation, 22* (3/4), 179-210.

Trovillo, P. V. (1939). A history of lie detection. *Criminology and Police Science, 29,* 848-881.

# Effects of Preparedness to Deceive on ERP Waveforms in a Two-Stimulus Paradigm

Jennifer M. C. Vendemia, PhD
Robert F. Buzan, MA
Eric P. Green, MA
Michael J. Schillaci, PhD

**SUMMARY.** Stimulus salience, attentional capture, and working memory load have all been theoretically and experimentally linked to deception (Allen & Iacono, 1997; Boaz, Perry, Raney, Fischler, & Shuman, 1991; Dionisio, Granholm, Hillix, & Perrine, 2001; Stelmack, Houlihan, & Doucet, 1994). This study manipulated working memory load by truthful and deceptive response demands combined with congruent and incongruent response demands. Response demands were randomly presented across trials requiring attention shifting within each trial, and preparedness to deceive was systematically decreased across three ex-

Jennifer M. C. Vendemia, Robert F. Buzan, Eric P. Green, and Michael J. Schillaci are affiliated with the Department of Psychology, University of South Carolina.

Address correspondence to: Jennifer M. C. Vendemia, Department of Psychology, University of South Carolina, Columbia, SC 29208 (E-mail: vendemia@mindspring.com).

The authors wish to acknowledge Dr. John Richards for his technical advice and support, and William Campbell for his aid in computer program design, testing participants, and data editing.

This research was supported by a grant from the Department of Defense Polygraph Institute, No. DABT60-00-1-1000, and a Major Research Instrumentation Award, No. BCS-9978198.

[Haworth co-indexing entry note]: "Effects of Preparedness to Deceive on ERP Waveforms in a Two-Stimulus Paradigm." Vendemia, Jennifer M. C., et al. Co-published simultaneously in *Journal of Neurotherapy* (The Haworth Medical Press, an imprint of The Haworth Press, Inc.) Vol. 9, No. 3, 2005, pp. 45-70; and: *Forensic Applications of QEEG and Neurotherapy* (ed: James R. Evans) The Haworth Medical Press, an imprint of The Haworth Press, Inc., 2005, pp. 45-70. Single or multiple copies of this article are available for a fee from The Haworth Document Delivery Service [1-800-HAWORTH, 9:00 a.m. - 5:00 p.m. (EST). E-mail address: docdelivery@haworthpress.com].

periments. Four waveforms were examined: an N2b occurring at 150-250 ms with an anterior maximum, a P3a occurring at 250-450 ms with an anterior maximum, an N4 occurring at 300-500 ms with an anterior and temporal maximum, and a P3b occurring at 500-700 ms with a parietal maximum. Results suggest that the processes of stimulus salience, attention shifting and resource allocation, long-term memory, and context updating are involved when individuals deceive. *[Article copies available for a fee from The Haworth Document Delivery Service: 1-800-HAWORTH. E-mail address: <docdelivery@haworthpress.com> Website: <http://www. HaworthPress.com> © 2005 by The Haworth Press, Inc. All rights reserved.]*

**KEYWORDS.** Deception, response congruity, ERP, preparedness

An individual's preparedness to tell a lie may have profound effects on any detection of deception methodology, including those that measure behavior, the peripheral nervous system, or the central nervous system. In real-world situations there are three common latencies between the onset of preparation to deceive and the lie itself. Individuals may prepare and rehearse a lie for days, weeks, or even years before they tell it. In some structured interview scenarios, such as a polygraph exam, they may have several minutes to prepare a response between the time the question is asked and their deceptive response. However, in most situations, such as witness interrogation or medical malingering, a question is asked and respondents must spontaneously evaluate that question, determine whether or not they wish to lie, and then prepare to make a truthful or deceptive response. This study examines the last category of questions.

We measured event-related brain potentials (ERPs), electroencephalographic signals time-linked to a cognitive activity, in three sequential experiments that systematically manipulated preparedness to deceive. ERP methodology allows researchers to evaluate the patterns of cortical activity associated with specific cognitive tasks; because all responses are temporally linked to specific stimuli or responses, we can say with certainty that any cortical activity measured was generated in response to given stimuli. As such, the current ERP-based paradigm allows us to form conclusions about differences in cortical activation patterns between truthful and deceptive responses and between respondents who are prepared to deceive and those who are not. Some participants were more prepared to respond deceptively or truthfully (i.e., received more information from Stimulus 1) than other participants based on the condition to which they were assigned. The ERP waveforms generated in each condition and across studies were analyzed to determine the impact of variations in preparedness.

ERPs have previously been used to examine the neurocognitive processes associated with deception. Conflicting cognitive theories of the processes underlying deception have been developed based on the mechanisms known to elicit these potentials. Theorists argue that the process of deception may involve attentional capture (Allen & Iacono, 1997), working memory load (Dionisio, Granholm, Hillix, & Perrine, 2001; Stelmack, Houlihan, & Doucet, 1994), or perceived incongruity with semantic and episodic memory (Boaz, Perry, Raney, Fischler, & Shuman, 1991). Regardless of theoretical approach, however, four ERP waveforms have been associated with deception, the P3b, P3a, N2b, and N4.

## *P3b*

The P300 (also known as the P3b), a large positive-going peak with a latency of 350-600 ms and a distribution whose maximum amplitude is at parietal sites and whose minimum amplitude is at anterior sites (Verleger, 1997), is by far the most frequently reported component of the four. It is typically studied in the context of the Concealed Information (CIT) oddball paradigm. This test consists of concealed information stimuli that occur infrequently eliciting a large P300, presented among a series of frequently occurring stimuli which do not involve concealed information and do not elicit a P300 (Allen, Iacono, & Danielson, 1992). When used in this type of paradigm, the P300 component of the ERP reliably and accurately indicates the presence of concealed knowledge (Allen & Iacono, 1997; Allen et al., 1992; Bashore & Rapp, 1993; Ellwanger, Rosenfeld, Sweet, & Bhatt, 1996; Farwell & Donchin, 1991; Rosenfeld, Ellwanger, & Sweet, 1995; Rosenfeld, Reinhart, & Bhatt, 1998; Rosenfeld, Sweet, Chuang, Ellwanger, & Song, 1996).

The spatio-temporal characteristics of the P300 observed in the CIT matches those of the P3b (Rosenfeld et al., 1999). The P3b is involved in many types of higher cortical functions including stimulus evaluation (Gevins, Cutillo, & Smith, 1995; Ruchkin, Johnson, Canoune, Ritter, & Hammer, 1990; Verleger, 1997), attention resource allocation (Comerchero & Polich, 1999), and updating of information held in working memory (Donchin & Coles, 1988; Ruchkin, Johnson, Canoune, & Ritter, 1990). Precisely which of these underlying processes are involved in deception is unclear, and in the CIT oddball task an often criticized confound of episodic memory further obscures interpretation (Allen & Iacono, 1997).

Because we removed the frequency related aspects of the task involved in a CIT that might impact the P300, we expected to see a suppression of the P300 amplitude related to the increased task demand of responding deceptively as opposed to truthfully. As the tasks became more difficult across experiments, we anticipated seeing greater suppression of the P3b across tasks.

## P3a

Like the P3b, the P3a is elicited by an oddball paradigm. The term "P3a" is applied to an assortment of early components with anterior distributions, and the exact conditions necessary to evoke a P3a vary across paradigm and stimulus demands (Katayama & Polich, 1998). In one variant of the oddball, the three-stimulus paradigm, the P3a occurs in response to novel-infrequent stimuli presented in addition to "typical" oddball stimuli. This waveform can also be elicited by shifts in attention (Comerchero & Polich, 1999), switching from difficult to easy task demands (Comerchero & Polich, 1999; Harmony et al., 2000), and alerting (Katayama & Polich, 1998). In general, the waveform is characterized as a positive-going peak with an anterior distribution and a latency of 250-350 ms (Comerchero & Polich, 1999; Harmony et al., 2000; Spencer, Dien, & Donchin, 1999). Two ERP studies of deception reported an early positivity with spatio-temporal characteristics similar to the P3a (Matsuda, Hira, Nakata, & Kakigi, 1990; Pollina & Squires, 1998). Neither study involved the oddball paradigm. In the current study, an equal-probability paradigm was used, thereby eliminating the probability confound. Therefore we expected to see a larger P3a related to attentional allocation for truthful responding, than related to attentional allocation for deceptive responding. As the P3a is related to attention switching between two levels of task difficulty such as deception vs. truth, but not related to overall task difficulty, we did not expect to see any differences between the waveforms related to the tasks.

## N2b

The N2b is elicited in attend conditions, and is associated with transient arousal and the orienting response (Loveless, 1983, 1986; Näätänen &

Gaillard, 1983). Therefore, decreased N2b latency is indicative of a lack of orienting toward task-related stimuli (Nordby, Hugdahl, Jasiukaitis, & Spiegal, 1999), and increased N2b latency is associated with the decline in attentional skill with age (Amenedio & Diaz, 1998). The N2b has also been associated with attention-switching tasks involving deception (Vendemia, 2003); individuals tend to orient to stimuli to which they must respond deceptively. We expected to see a larger N2b related to deceptive responses than truthful responses. As the tasks became more difficult and the response prompt became more relevant to the correct completion of the task, we expected to see greater N2b waveforms.

## N4

The N4 component, a large negative-going peak at around 400 ms with maximum amplitude in anterior and temporal regions, is sensitive to semantic incongruity (such as in the sentence, "This morning for breakfast I had a nice hot cup of whiskers"). Researchers argue that deception represents an incongruity between internal truth and external response (Bashore & Rapp, 1993). The N4 has been elicited by the possession of concealed knowledge in tasks involving false sentence completions (Boaz et al., 1991) and in a two-stimulus target detection task (Matsuda et al., 1990). Bashore and Rapp (1993) suggest that the N4 is reactive to anomalies in semantic and episodic memory as well as to inconsistencies in language semantics. In a two-stimulus task, the N4 was not found to be sensitive to deception, but was sensitive to response congruity with the second stimulus (Stelmack, Houlihan, & Doucet, 1994; Stelmack, Houlihan, Doucet, & Belisle, 1994).

The current study used a two-stimulus paradigm in which the first stimulus consisted of a statement and the second of a "true" or "false" prompt. Similar to studies by Stelmack and colleagues (Stelmack, Houlihan, & Doucet, 1994; Stelmack, Houlihan, Doucet, & Belisle, 1994), participants were asked to evaluate the first stimulus and, based on its truth-value, agree or disagree with the second stimulus. The paradigm was based on the Directed Lie Test (DLT), which is a reliable and valid measure of deception (Honts & Raskin, 1988; Raskin, Kircher, Horowitz, & Honts, 1989). In the DLT, participants are instructed to tell lies to specific questions, such as responding "No" to the question, "Have you ever exceeded the speed limit?"

The paradigm was designed to control for a number the factors known to affect ERP signals. Attentional capture was manipulated by the use of an attention-switching paradigm, while multiple levels of task difficulty assessed working memory load. Using sentence evaluation instead of denial of recall-based information eliminated the issue of episodic memory. Additionally, the equiprobable nature and random presentation of the deceptive and truthful conditions allowed the effects of attention and workload to be parametrically equated on a trial-by-trial basis independent of stimulus presentation probability, which controls for and eliminates potential probability confounds.

Because we used an attention-switching paradigm, a P3a was expected. In addition, we expected that the amplitude of both the P3a and P3b would be suppressed for deceptive responses relative to truthful responses because of the increased task demand of responding deceptively as opposed to truthfully (Pollina & Squires, 1998; Vendemia, 2003). Based on previous findings (Vendemia, 2003), we hypothesized an increased latency of the N2b in deceptive conditions relative to truthful conditions. However, evidence from the same study suggesting that the N4 is not correlated with deception led us to predict that the N4 would not discriminate between deceptive and truthful conditions, but that it would be affected by congruity.

We expected that reduced preparedness to deceive would increase the salience of Stimulus 2. As the salience of this stimulus item increased, so too would attentional resource allocation. The ERP effects of this, we hypothesized, would be suppressed P3a amplitude (Wilson, Swain, & Ullsperger, 1998) and increased P3b amplitude (McGarry-Roberts, Stelmack, & Campbell, 1992; Picton, 1992; Kok, 2001; Vendemia, 2003). Based on as yet unpublished results in our laboratory, we expected P3a and P3b latencies to decrease with increasing preparedness to deceive.

## METHOD

Three studies of increasing difficulty were conducted to examine ERP waveforms in relation to deception, response congruity, and preparedness to deceive. Participants were asked to evaluate sentences (Stimulus 1) that were either true or false, compare those evaluations with a second stimulus (Stimulus 2; either "true" or "false"), and respond truthfully or deceptively. In Experiment 1, all the information needed for participants to correctly complete the task was presented within Stimulus 1. That is, both congruity and deception (BCD) were predictable from Stimulus 1. In Experiment 2, information regarding deception was available from the first stimulus, but information regarding response congruity was not available until the onset of Stimulus 2. That is, only deception (OD) was predictable from Stimulus 1. Experiment 3 reduced the predictive value of Stimulus 1 to zero (i.e., neither congruity nor deception were predictable; NCD), increasing the amount of information to be absorbed from Stimulus 2. This resulted in greater salience and workload demands across the experiments, as shown in Table 1.

### Experiment 1

*Participants.* Participants were 34 undergraduate students recruited from the University of South Carolina student population. Demographics for all three experiments are given in Table 2. All were right handed and had normal or corrected to normal vision with no known color impairments. Participants were also screened for a variety of neurological and medical disorders and were asked to avoid drugs, alcohol, and caffeine for 24 hours preceding the experiment. Participants received course credit for their participation.

*Task.* Each participant sat in a comfortable chair approximately 122 cm from a 29-inch color video computer monitor (NEC Multisync XM29) displaying at 1280 horizontal and 1024 vertical pixels.

The two-stimulus paradigm involved the pairing of a first stimulus, a statement which participants evaluated, and a second stimulus ("true" or "false") to which they responded. Each first stimulus was drawn from a series of 60 sentences involving declarative knowledge that were designed to be easily verified as true or false (e.g., "I am human"). Several examples of the sentences used are shown in Table 3. These stimuli were derived from a set of 100 short, easy to understand sentences that had been pre-tested with an undergraduate sample at the University. Raters were asked to decide whether each sentence was true or false. Only those items unanimously rated as "true" or "false" during pre-testing were retained for the experiments.

Sentence presentation lasted 2500 ms, followed by a 750 ms fixation point, then a second stimulus of 2500 ms duration (see Table 1). Participants responded to the second stimulus by pressing a key to indicate whether it agreed or disagreed with their answer to the first stimulus. This procedure is similar in nature to that used by Rosenfeld et al. (1996), a modified forced-choice procedure to detect malingering.

Participants were required to make a congruent response (i.e., "agree") on 50% of the trials and an incongruent response (i.e., "disagree") on the other 50% of the trials. Additionally, participants were cued by stim-

TABLE 1. Experimental Procedure, Stimulus 1 Predictability, and Anticipated Responses

| Experiment/Condition | Stimulus 1 (2500 ms) | Fixation (750 ms) | Stimulus 2 (2500 ms) | Correct Response |
|---|---|---|---|---|
| **Experiment 1 (BCD)** | Predicts deception and congruity | | | |
| Congruent Truthful | The grass is red | + | False | Agree |
| Congruent Deceptive | **The grass is red** | + | True | Agree |
| Incongruent Truthful | The grass is green | + | False | Disagree |
| Incongruent Deceptive | **The grass is green** | + | True | Disagree |
| **Experiment 2 (OD)** | | | | |
| Base True | Predicts deception | | | |
| Congruent Truthful | The grass is green | + | True | Agree |
| Congruent Deceptive | The grass is green | + | False | Agree |
| Incongruent Truthful | The grass is green | + | False | Disagree |
| Incongruent Deceptive | The grass is green | + | True | Disagree |
| Base False | | | | |
| Congruent Truthful | The grass is red | + | False | Agree |
| Congruent Deceptive | The grass is red | + | True | Agree |
| Incongruent Truthful | The grass is red | + | True | Disagree |
| Incongruent Deceptive | The grass is red | + | False | Disagree |
| **Experiment 3 (NCD)** | Predicts nothing | | | |
| Base True | | | | |
| Congruent Truthful | The grass is green | + | True | Agree |
| Congruent Deceptive | The grass is green | + | False | Agree |
| Incongruent Truthful | The grass is green | + | False | Disagree |
| Incongruent Deceptive | The grass is green | + | True | Disagree |
| Base False | | | | |
| Congruent Truthful | The grass is red | + | False | Agree |
| Congruent Deceptive | The grass is red | + | True | Agree |
| Incongruent Truthful | The grass is red | + | True | Disagree |
| Incongruent Deceptive | The grass is red | + | False | Disagree |

Note. In this example, *BLUE* text cues the participant to respond truthfully, while **RED** text cues the participant to respond deceptively. This designation was counterbalanced throughout the experiments. The key difference between Experiments 1 and 2 is that in Experiment 1 Stimulus 1 predicts both deception and congruity, whereas Stimulus 1 in Experiment 2 predicts only deception. Unlike the first stimulus in Experiment 1, the first stimulus in Experiment 2 (e.g., "The grass is green") could be followed by a Stimulus 2 value of "True" or "False," thus changing the correct response. Therefore, Stimulus 1 does not predict congruity.

TABLE 2. Demographic Information for Participants Across the Three Studies (n = 84)

| | Sex | | Age | | |
| --- | --- | --- | --- | --- | --- |
| | Men (n) | Women (n) | Range | M | SD |
| Experiment 1 (n = 34) | 19 | 15 | 18-39 | 21 | 4.09 |
| Experiment 2 (n = 27) | 11 | 16 | 18-24 | 20 | 1.89 |
| Experiment 3 (n = 23) | 8 | 15 | 18-25 | 20 | 1.85 |
| Total (n = 84) | 38 | 46 | 18-39 | 20 | 3.05 |

TABLE 3. Examples of Sentences Used in the Three Experiments

| Base Truth Value | Stimulus Sentence |
| --- | --- |
| True | The grass is green. |
| | South Carolina is in the United States. |
| | Ducks spend most of their time in the water. |
| | A piano is a musical instrument. |
| | Poodles are dogs. |
| False | Snakes have 13 legs. |
| | People are born wearing clothes. |
| | The slowest runner always wins the race. |
| | Cupcakes are healthier than salad. |
| | President George Washington cleans my kitchen. |

ulus color to respond deceptively on 50% of the trials and truthfully on the other 50%. The stimuli were presented in red or blue. Participants were randomly assigned color cued deception. Deceptive and truthful trials were randomly presented. Furthermore, the color of Stimulus 1 always predicted Stimulus 2 (i.e., the color of Stimulus 1 always matched the color of Stimulus 2). Thus, both congruity and deception (BCD) were predictable from Stimulus 1–the defining feature of Experiment 1. For example, when presented with a red Stimulus 1, a given participant would always receive a red "true" as Stimulus 2. The relationship between color and Stimulus 2 was counterbalanced across participants.

As shown in Table 1, when participants were color cued to be truthful and the second stimulus provided an accurate description of the truth state of the first stimulus, they responded by pressing "agree." We labeled this "congruent truthful" to denote that the respondent truthfully indicated that the second stimulus was congruent with their answer to the first stimulus. When color cued to be truthful and the second stimulus did not provide an accurate assessment of the truth state of the first stimulus, they responded by pressing "disagree" (incongruent truthful). When color cued to be deceptive and the second stimulus provided an inaccurate answer, they responded "agree" (congruent lie). Finally, when color cued to be deceptive but the second stimulus accurately described the truth state of Stimulus 1, they responded "disagree" (incongruent lie). This resulted in four experimental conditions: congruent truthful, congruent lie, incongruent truthful and incongruent lie (CT, CL, IT, IL). ERP data were collected on three blocks of 60 randomized trials each. This resulted in 45 trials of each trial type.

*Procedure.* Participants arrived at the lab on the day of the experiment and were familiarized with the research procedure before signing the consent form. They practiced on a pencil and paper measure that included all stimuli used in the study. Following the paper task, participants were seated in front of the monitor, verbally instructed on the use of the response box, and received additional computer-based practice to train them to respond within the allowed response window of 2500 ms. The computer-based practice consisted of 12 items from the larger block of questions, constrained so that it contained equal numbers of CL, CT, IL, and IT questions. Participants were required to attain a 67% accuracy level on each of the trial types in order to begin the experiment. Records of the number of practice block repetitions required and the time to completion were not kept, but six participants were disqualified from further participation because they could not achieve the 67% correct threshold. During the experiment, participants initiated each trial by key press. They were instructed to rest during the period between trials if they felt tired. During the rest period, the stimulus presentation screen reminded participants of the response box instructions.

## Experiment 2

In the second study, response congruity was not predictable from cues in Stimulus 1. In other words, Stimulus 1 was colored either red or blue, but Stimulus 2 did not predict congruity. Thus, participants could utilize the color of Stimulus 1 to prepare to lie or tell the truth, but could not predict whether they would do so by agreeing or disagreeing.

*Participants.* Participants were 27 undergraduate students (see Table 2) recruited using the same procedures as in Experiment 1.

*Task.* The task was identical to the task in Experiment 1 with one exception. In the second study, the first stimulus only predicted deception, not response congruity. Thus, participants would not be able to determine the specific response until the onset of the second stimulus. As in all three experiments, deception cue color was randomly assigned.

*Procedure.* The procedure was identical to Experiment 1.

## Experiment 3

In the third study, Stimulus 1 sentences were colored black, offering no predictive value for either response congruity or the truth-value of the response. Participants could prepare neither to respond deceptively or truthfully nor to agree or disagree in response to the stimuli.

*Participants.* Participants were 23 undergraduate students (see Table 2) recruited using the same procedures as in Experiment 1.

*Task.* The task in Experiment 3 differed from the task in the earlier experiments in two ways. In the first study, the first stimulus predicted both deception and response. In the second study, the first stimulus only predicted deception. In the third study, the first stimulus predicted neither deception nor congruity (see Table 1). Thus, participants would not be able to predict the nature of the response until the onset of the second stimulus. In addition, the presentation time of the second stimulus was increased to 3000 ms to allow participants enough time to respond. This modification was based on pilot testing, which indicated that participants in this more difficult experiment required more time to generate the correct response.

*Procedure.* The procedure was identical to Experiments 1 and 2.

*Recording and Segmenting of EEG for ERP.* ERPs in truthful and deceptive conditions were recorded using a 128 channel "Geodesic Sensor Net" with the EGI system (Electrical Geodesics, Inc., Eugene, OR; Tucker, Liotti, Potts, Russell, & Posner, 1994). The net was positioned according to its anatomically marked locations. Sites on this cap can be interpolated to those of the International 10-20 system (Luu & Ferree, 2000; Srinivasan, Tucker, & Murias, 1998). The signal was referenced to the vertex. Impedances were kept below 100 k$\Omega$, and the signal was amplified with the EGI "NetAmps" that consist of high-impedance amplifiers and a PowerPC-based computer system. The EGI "NetStation" computer program was used to control zero and gain calibrations for each participant, impedance calibration, A/D sampling (250 Hz), and

EEG data storage. Band-pass filters were set at 0.1 to 100 Hz with 20K amplification.

A second computer was time-synchronized with the PowerPC running the NetStation computer program so that time and trial information was stored with the EEG recordings. The data were segmented offline using a 600 ms baseline and 1000 ms post-stimulus period. Electrodes that exceeded a 70 μV threshold were eliminated from further analysis. Trials that contained more than 10 "bad" electrodes, an eye blink, or an incorrect response to the second stimulus were eliminated. The cut-off 10 "bad" electrodes (7.7% of the total electrodes), were 2.7% more of the data than the 5% total bad electrode limit suggested by Picton et al., (2000). However, in line with their suggestions, electrodes up to the 7.7% cut-off were interpolated using spherical splines. After this stage of data analysis any participant with more than 20 trials (11%) of the experimental trials rejected for any reason were eliminated from further analyses. This strategy was based on the minimum number of trials necessary to develop an observable ERP from the averaged data. Five of the original 84 participants were eliminated through these procedures. For the rest of the participants missing data were replaced using the averaged potential of the five closest electrodes. Data were re-referenced to a mastoid reference offline, baseline corrected using the 100 ms pre-stimulus interval and filtered from 1 to 30 Hz.

## RESULTS

A series of $2 \times 2 \times 3$ mixed measures ANOVAs (Deception $\times$ Congruity $\times$ Predictability) compared the amplitudes and latencies of four waveforms (i.e., N4, N2b, P3a, and P3b) across regions specific to the distribution of each waveform (see Figure 1). All significant tests were followed with appropriate post-hoc analyses, and only significant findings are reported. Figure 2 shows a sample topographic distribution for each waveform. Waveforms were identified according to the following pre-selected windows: N4, 300-500 ms; N2b, 150-250 ms; P3a, 250-450 ms; P3b, 500-700 ms. Findings will be discussed relative to predictability condition: Experiment 1–both congruity and deception predictable (BCD), Experiment 2–only deception predictable (OD), and Experiment 3–neither deception nor congruity predictable (NCD).

FIGURE 1. Eighteen regions of 6 averaged electrodes each based on the 10-20 system. FL, FM, FR, FCL, and FCR represents frontal left, middle, right, central left, and central right. TLA, TLP, TRA, and TRP represents temporal, left anterior, left posterior, right anterior and right posterior. CL, CM, and CR represents central left middle and right; PL, PM, and PR represents parietal left, middle, and right, and OL, OM, and OR represent occipital left, middle, and right.

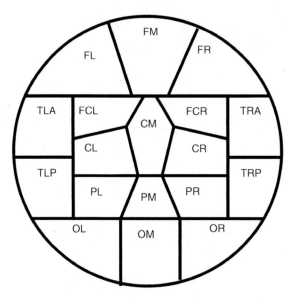

## N2b

Mixed ANOVAs for the N2b amplitude and latency were conducted on anterior temporal, frontal, and central regions–the regions specific to the distribution of the N2b. There was a main effect of predictability at the left anterior region such that N2b latencies were longest in the NCD condition and shortest in the BCD condition [$F(2, 81) = 3.38, p = .04, \eta^2 = .08$].

There were significant latency two-way interactions between predictability and deception in the left frontal [$F(2,81) = 3.27, p = 0.04, \eta^2 = .08$] and left central [$F(2,81) = 3.99, p = 0.02, \eta^2 = 0.09$] regions. As can be seen in Figure 3, N2b latencies for truthful and deceptive responses were not significantly different in BCD. In OD at the left frontal region there was a trend towards N2b latency being longer for truthful than deceptive responses. In the left central region in BCD and OD the N2b la-

FIGURE 2. Illustrative topographic distributions for the N2b (CT, OD), P3a (IL, OD), P3b (IL, 2200), and N4 (CL, NCD).

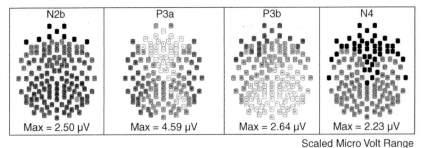

tency did not differ between response types, but in NCD the latency for truthful responses was longer than for deceptive responses.

## *P3a*

Mixed ANOVAs for the P3a were conducted in the frontal and central regions. As Figure 4 shows, in the middle central region, the amplitude of the P3a was greater when participants responded truthfully $F(1, 81) = 8.59, p = .005, \eta^2 = .11$. In the frontocentral central region, there was a trend for the latency of the P3a to be shorter for truthful responses (M = 378.94 ms, SE = 1.91), than for deceptive responses [$M = 383.61, SE = 1.86; F(1,81) = 3.83, p = .054, \eta^2 = .05$]. In the right frontocentral region, the latency of the P3a differed with predictability $F(2,81) = 3.35, p = .041, \eta^2 = .05$ such that the latency of the P3a was longest for the OD group and shortest for the BCD group.

There were no two-way interactions, but a three-way interaction occurred in the right frontocentral region [$F(2,81) = 4.02, p = .022, \eta^2 = .11$]. As seen in Figure 5, the latency of truthful responses was longer than deceptive response in the BCD group. In the OD group, truthful responses were associated with a longer P3a latency than deceptive responses only when participants agreed, while in the NCD group truthful responses had a longer latency than deceptive responses only when participants disagreed.

FIGURE 3. Latency of the N2b for truthful and deceptive responses at left frontal and left central regions for the BCD, OD, and NCD groups.

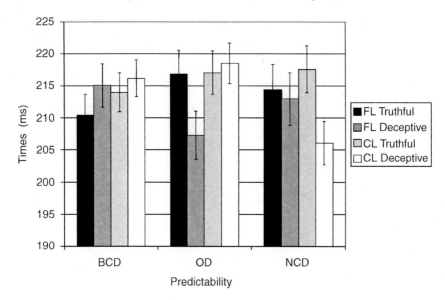

## P3b

Mixed ANOVAs for the P3b were conducted for the parietal, central, and frontocentral regions. Waveforms for all conditions are shown at the parietal region in Figure 6.

In the frontocentral region, the P3b amplitude for deceptive responses ($M = 2.59$, $SE = 0.18$) was significantly smaller than for truthful responses [$M = 2.75$, $SE = 0.19$; $F(1,81) = 4.23$, $p = 0.04$, $\eta^2 = 0.05$].

Across central and parietal regions, P3b amplitude was greater when participants agreed than when they disagreed, as shown in Table 4. The magnitude of this difference was largest in the mid-parietal region ($M = 3.34$ μV, $SE = .23$ vs. $M = 2.93$ μV, $SE = .20$). P3b latency in these regions was longer when participants agreed than when they disagreed, and this difference was similarly largest in the mid-parietal region ($M = 655.81$ ms, $SE = 3.84$ vs. $M = 629.99$ ms, $SE = 4.62$ ms).

There were three-way interactions involving the latency of the P3b in the middle and right central and parietal regions (Table 4). The latency difference between truthful responses and deceptive responses remained constant between BCD and OD conditions for both agree and dis-

FIGURE 4. Waveforms for truthful vs. deceptive responses at the middle central region for all participants (n = 81).

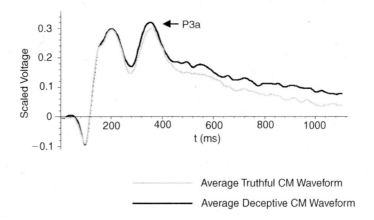

agree responses. In the NCD condition, however, the latency difference increased when participants agreed and decreased when they disagreed (see Figure 7).

## N4

Mixed ANOVAs on N4 latency and amplitude were conducted for the anterior temporal, frontal, and central regions (Table 5). Anterior Temporal N4 waveforms for all conditions are shown in Figure 8. There were main effects for deception in the right and left anterior temporal regions. In the right anterior temporal region, the amplitude for truthful responses ($M = -1.40$ µV, $SE = 0.06$) was larger than for deceptive responses ($M = -1.27$ µV, $SE = 0.05$). In the left anterior temporal region, the latency for truthful responses ($M = 443.42$, SE = 3.41) was shorter than for deceptive responses ($M = 450.91$, $SE = 3.35$).

There were interactions between congruity and deception for amplitude at the left and right frontocentral regions, right central region, and right posterior temporal region. As can be seen in Figure 8 (showing anterior temporal regions), the amplitude for IL was larger than IT in all regions, and CL amplitude was larger than CT amplitude in most regions. There were also two-way interactions for latency in the frontocentral and left central regions such that the latency for deceptive responses was greater than for truthful responses, and the difference in latency was much smaller for disagree than agree responses.

FIGURE 5. Event-related waveform at right frontal sites between all four response types for BCD, OD, and NCD groups.

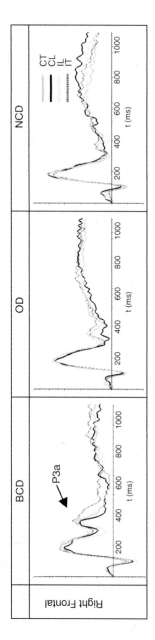

FIGURE 6. Event-related waveform at right frontal sites between all four response types for BCD, OD, and NCD groups..

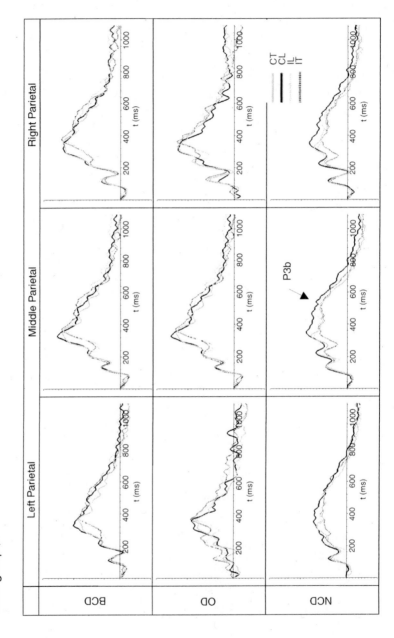

FIGURE 7. The difference in P3b latency between truthful and deceptive responses when participants responded by agreeing and disagreeing across levels of predictability.

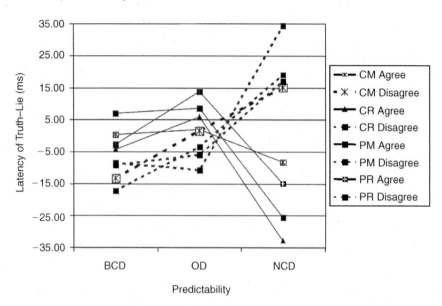

There was an interaction in N4 latency between deception and predictability at the left temporal region such that the latency for truthful responses was smaller than for deceptive responses in the BCD and NCD conditions, but there was no difference in the OD condition.

## DISCUSSION

### Deception

As expected, the amplitude of the P3a was larger when participants responded truthfully as compared to deceptively. This is consistent with Comerchero and Polich's (1998) attention switching theory of the P3a, which suggests that the amplitude of the P3a is increased when individuals switch from more difficult to easier task demands. Additionally, we found that deception suppressed the amplitude of the P3b waveform regardless of preparedness to deceive. This is consistent with previous findings (Stelmack, Houlihan, & Doucet, 1994; Stelmack, Houlihan,

TABLE 4. Significant ANOVA Results (con × dec × pred) for the Amplitude and Latency of the P3b Waveform

| Source | df | F | $\eta^2$ | p |
|---|---|---|---|---|
| Amplitude | | | | |
| FCL (dec) | 1 | 4.23 | 0.05 | 0.04 |
| PL (con) | 1 | 5.39 | 0.06 | 0.02 |
| CL (con) | 1 | 9.76 | 0.11 | 0.00 |
| CR (con) | 1 | 17.56 | 0.18 | 0.00 |
| CM (con) | 1 | 12.57 | 0.13 | 0.00 |
| PM (con) | 1 | 10.44 | 0.11 | 0.00 |
| PR (con) | 1 | 9.16 | 0.10 | 0.00 |
| FCR (con × dec) | 1 | 5.70 | 0.07 | 0.02 |
| FCL (con × pred) | 2 | 3.63 | 0.08 | 0.03 |
| CL (dec × pred) | 2 | 3.60 | 0.08 | 0.03 |
| Latency | | | | |
| PL (con) | 1 | 14.58 | 0.15 | 0.00 |
| PM (con) | 1 | 46.90 | 0.37 | 0.00 |
| PR (con) | 1 | 28.96 | 0.26 | 0.00 |
| CR (con) | 1 | 43.50 | 0.35 | 0.00 |
| CR (pred) | 2 | 3.33 | 0.08 | 0.04 |
| PL (con × dec × pred) | 2 | 6.00 | 0.13 | 0.00 |
| PM (con × dec × pred) | 2 | 11.23 | 0.22 | 0.00 |
| PR (con × dec × pred) | 2 | 4.20 | 0.09 | 0.02 |
| CR (con × dec × pred) | 2 | 12.18 | 0.23 | 0.00 |

*Note.* Condition abbreviations: Con = Congruity, Dec = Deception, Pred = Prediction. Error *df* = 81.

Doucet, & Belisle, 1994; Vendemia, 2003) and suggests that deception is cognitively challenging no matter how prepared the respondent is to deceive.

Deception also suppressed the N4 amplitude, contrary to our predictions. While it is believed that the N4 is related to semantic incongruity, it has been elicited by the possession of concealed knowledge in sentence completion tasks involving false sentence completions (Boaz et al., 1991) and in a two-stimulus target detection task (Matsuda et al., 1990). One can conceive of deception as an incongruity between the internal truth and the external response (Bashore & Rapp, 1993), an interpretation that is supported by this finding.

TABLE 5. Significant ANOVA Results (con × dec × pred) for the Amplitude and Latency of the N4 Waveform

| Source | df | F | $\eta^2$ | p |
|---|---|---|---|---|
| Amplitude | | | | |
| TRA (dec) | 1 | 5.32 | 0.06 | 0.02 |
| FCL (con × pred) | 2 | 4.67 | 0.10 | 0.01 |
| FCR (con × dec) | 1 | 5.12 | 0.06 | 0.03 |
| TRP (con × dec) | 1 | 4.08 | 0.05 | 0.05 |
| CR (con × dec) | 1 | 6.63 | 0.04 | 0.18 |
| CM (con × dec × pred) | 2 | 4.19 | 0.09 | 0.02 |
| Latency | | | | |
| TLA (dec) | 1 | 7.35 | 0.08 | 0.01 |
| FCL (con × pred) | 2 | 5.35 | 0.12 | 0.01 |
| CL (con × pred) | 2 | 5.56 | 0.12 | 0.01 |
| TLA (dec × pred) | 2 | 4.43 | 0.10 | 0.02 |

*Note.* Condition abbreviations: Con = Congruity, Dec = Deception, Pred = Prediction. Error *df* = 81.

## Congruity

Significant main effects were found for the effect of response congruity on the centrally- and parietally-generated P3b, such that P3b amplitude was suppressed and the latency was generally decreased for incongruous responses versus congruous responses. The same effect was found for the N2b in mid and right parietal and occipital regions.

## Predictability

As predicted, reduced preparedness to deceive led to suppressed P3a amplitude and decreased P3a latency. We also found that decreasing predictability led to shorter P3b latencies. However, contrary to our predictions, we found that as predictability decreased, P3b amplitude increased and N2b latency increased. These findings suggest that reducing preparedness to deceive does in fact increase the salience of the Stimulus 2 in the two-stimulus paradigm. As more information must be drawn from this stimulus, the attentional resources allocated to it must necessarily increase, as indicated by the effects of predictability on the P3a. Concurrent with or following this period of focused attention, the participant must orient to the information presented in the second stimulus, a task made more important as preparedness to deceive decreases. This is reflected in the variations in N2b latency, which increased as predictability decreased. Just as the act of formulating a deceptive response is more cognitively challenging than generating a truthful response, so too is generating any response with decreasing preparedness. That is, as participants receive less information from Stimulus 1, more information must be gleaned from Stimulus 2, a decision to deceive or tell the truth must be made, an answer formulated, and a response completed.

## CONCLUSIONS

Previous theories of deceptive responding have postulated attention, working memory load, and congruity as sources of ERP variation between deception and truth. This study suggests that processes related to all three theories underlie deception. Particularly when studying brain waves associated with deception, it is extremely important to control for variables that may affect salience and workload, as these two processes have conflicting effects on ERPs, particularly the P3b.

Individuals in each experiment shifted their attention to allocate resources to specific task demands, which themselves exerted separate effects for deception and congruity. The P3a, with neuronal sources in the anterior cingulate, seems to result from orienting towards task-related stimuli, such as congruity and deception (Vendemia, 2003). It is possible that the inherent incongruity of deception is also attended to at this time, reflected in the effects of deception on the P3a.

Following that initial attentional response, additional processing of congruity occurs across multiple regions of the frontal and temporal lobes, affecting the N4. The subsequent P3b engages decision-making processes and response selection. Workload associated with the additive effects of deception and congruity also suppressed the amplitude of the P3b, but as the salience of the second stimulus increased the pattern of amplitude suppression became less defined. Stimulus salience, manipulated by predictability, exerted a generalized impact on the N2b. The pattern of the N2b, related to stimulus salience, the P3a, related to orienting and attention shifting, the N4 related to comparison with internal semantic truth, and P3b related to ongoing workload and decision form a series of processes that are involved in deceptive processing.

FIGURE 8. Event-related waveforms in the left and right anterior temporal regions between all four response types for BCD, OD, and NCD groups.

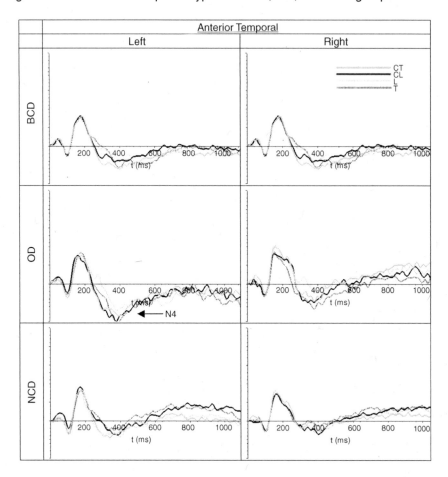

We would anticipate that these findings are potentially useful in a variety of settings in which deception could occur. Because of the flexibility inherent in ERP-based paradigms, this methodology has possible applications in criminal investigations, terrorism prevention, and the detection of clinical malingering. Vendemia and Buzan (2004) utilized a similar two-stimulus paradigm to successfully identify more than 86% of "guilty" participants in a mock-crime experiment. Question sets can also be designed to evaluate terrorism-related guilt: connections to known terrorists, details of possible attacks, or involvement in past, present, or future terrorist plots. In clinical practice, questions can be formulated to detect patient attempts to fake the results of their evaluations. However, it should be noted that this methodology is not sufficiently developed for clinical use; data analysis is currently extremely time-intensive, taking up to a week to detect deception. With ongoing research, we expect to develop more real-time analysis tools that will provide clinicians with a quick and accurate tool to detect malingering within the time constraints of a medical or psychological evaluation.

# REFERENCES

Allen, J. J., & Iacono, W. G. (1997). A comparison of methods for the analysis of event-related potentials in deception detection. *Psychophysiology, 34*, 234-240.

Allen, J. J., Iacono, W. G., & Danielson, K. D. (1992). The identification of concealed memories using the event-related potential and implicit behavioral measures: A methodology for prediction in the face of individual differences. *Psychophysiology, 29*, 504-522.

Amenedo, E., & Diaz, F. (1998). Automatic and effortful processes in auditory memory reflected by event-related potentials: Age related findings. *Electroencephalography and Clinical Neurophysiology: Evoked Potentials, 108*, 361-369.

Bashore, T. R., & Rapp, P. E. (1993). Are there alternatives to traditional polygraph procedures? *Psychological Bulletin, 113*, 3-22.

Boaz, T. L., Perry, N. W., Raney, G., Fischler, I. S., & Shuman, D. (1991). Detection of guilty knowledge with event-related potentials. *Journal of Applied Psychology, 76*, 788-795.

Comerchero M. D., & Polich, J. (1999). P3a and P3b from typical auditory and visual stimuli. *Clinical Neurophysiology, 110*, 24-30.

Department of Defense Polygraph Institute. (2003). *Neural mechanisms of deception and response congruity to general knowledge information and autobiographical information in visual two-stimulus paradigms with motor response* (Publication No. DoDPI99-P-0010).

Dionisio, D. P., Granholm, E., Hillix, W. A., & Perrine, W. F. (2001). Differentiation of deception using pupillary response as an index of cognitive processing. *Psychophysiology, 38*, 205-211.

Donchin, E., & Coles, M. G. H. (1988). Is the P300 a manifestation of context updating? *Behavioral and Brain Sciences, 121*, 357-374.

Ellwanger, J., Rosenfeld, J. P., Sweet, J. J., & Bhatt, M. (1996). Detecting simulated amnesia for autobiographical and recently learned information using the P300 event-related potential. *International Journal of Psychophysiology, 23*, 9-23.

Farwell, L. A., & Donchin, E. (1991). The truth will out: Interrogative polygraphy ("lie detection") with event-related brain potentials. *Psychophysiology, 28*, 531-547.

Gevins, A., Cutillo, B., & Smith, M. E., (1995). Regional modulation of high resolution evoked potentials during verbal and non-verbal matching tasks. *Electroencephalography and Clinical Neurophysiology, 94*, 129-147.

Harmony, T., Bernal., J., Fernández, T., T., Silva-Pereyra, J., Fernández-Bouzas, A., Marosi, R., et al. (2000). Primary task demands modulate P3 amplitude. *Cognitive Brain Research, 9*, 53-60.

Honts, C. R., & Raskin, D. C. (1988). A field study of the validity of the directed lie control question. *Journal of Police Science and Administration, 16*, 56-61.

Katayama, J., & Polich, J. (1998). Stimulus context determines P3a and P3b. *Psychophysiology, 35*, 23-33.

Kok, A. (2001). On the utility of P3 amplitude as a measure of processing capacity. *Psychophysiology, 39*, 557-577.

Loveless, N. E. (1983). The orienting response and evoked potentials in man. In D. Siddle (Ed.), *Orienting and habituation: Perspectives in human research.* (pp. 71-108). New York: Wiley.

Loveless, N. E. (1986). Potentials evoked by temporal deviance. *Biological Psychology, 22*, 149-167.

Luu, P., & Ferree, T. (2000). *Determination of the Geodesic Densor Nets' electrode positions and their 10-10 international equivalents.* [Technical Note]. Eugene, OR: Electrical Geodesics Incorporated.

Matsuda, T., Hira, S, Nakata, M., & Kakigi, S. (1990). The effect of one's own name upon event related potentials: Event related (P3 and CNV) as an index of deception. *Japanese Journal of Physiological Psychology and Psychophysiology, 8*, 9-18.

McGarry-Roberts, P. A., Stelmack, R. M., & Campbell, K. B. (1992). Intelligence, reaction time, and event-related potentials. *Intelligence, 16*, 289-313.

Näätänen, R., & Gaillard, A. W. K. (1983). The N2 deflection of ERP and the orienting reflex. In A.W.K. Gaillard & W. Ritter (Eds.), *EEG correlates of information processing: Theoretical issues* (pp. 119-141). Amsterdam: North Holland.

Nordby, H., Hugdahl, K., Jasiukaitis, P., & Spiegal, D. (1999). Effects of hypnotizability on performance of a Stroop task and event related potentials. *Perceptual and Motor Skills, 88*, 818-830.

Picton, T. W. (1992). The P300 wave of the human event-related potential. *Journal of Clinical Neurophysiology, 9*, 456-479.

Picton, T.W., Bentin, S., Berg, P., Donchin, E., Hillyard, S. A., Johnson, R., Jr., et al. (2000). Committee Report: Guidelines for using human event-related potentials to study cognition: Recording standards and publication criteria. *Psychophysiology, 37*, 127-152.

Pollina, D. A., & Squires, N. K. (1998). Many-valued logic and event-related potentials. *Brain and Language, 63*, 321-345.

Raskin, D. C., Kircher, J. C., Horowitz, S. W., & Honts, C. R. (1989). Recent laboratory and field research on polygraph techniques. In J. C. Yuille (Ed.), *Credibility assessment* (pp. 1-24). London: Kluwer Academic Publishers.

Rosenfeld, J. P., Ellwanger, J. W., Nolan, K., Wu, S., Bermann, R. G., & Sweet, J. (1999). P300 scalp amplitude distribution as an index of deception in a simulated cognitive deficit model. *International Journal of Psychophysiology, 33*, 3-19.

Rosenfeld, J. P., Ellwanger, J., & Sweet, J. (1995). Detecting simulated amnesia with event-related brain potentials. *International Journal of Psychophysiology, 19*, 1-11.

Rosenfeld, J. P., Reinhart, A. M., & Bhatt, M. (1998). P300 correlates of simulated malingered amnesia in a matching-to-sample task: Topographic analyses of deception versus truthtelling responses. *International Journal of Psychophysiology, 28,* 233-247.

Rosenfeld, J. P., Sweet, J. J., Chuang, J., Ellwanger, J., & Song, L. (1996). Detection of simulated malingering using forced choice recognition enhanced with event-related potential recording. *The Clinical Neuropsychologist, 10,* 163-179.

Ruchkin, D. S., Johnson, R., Canoune, H. L., & Ritter, W. (1990). Short-term memory storage and retention: An event-related brain potential study. *Electroencephalography and Clinical Neurophysiology, 76,* 419-439.

Ruchkin, D. S., Johnson, R., Canoune, H. L., Ritter, W., & Hammer, M. (1990). Multiple sources of the P3b associated with different types of information. *Psychophysiology, 27,* 157-176.

Spencer, K. M., Dien, J., & Donchin, E. (1999). A componential analysis of the ERP elicited by novel events using a dense electrode array. *Psychophysiology, 36,* 409-414.

Srinivasan, R., Tucker, D. M., & Murias, M. (1998). Estimated the spatial Nyquist of the human EEG. *Behavioral Research Methods, Instruments, & Computers, 30,* 8-19.

Stelmack, R. M., Houlihan, M., & Doucet, C. (1994). *Event-related potentials and the detection of deception: A two-stimulus paradigm.* Ottawa: University of Ottawa. (NTIS No. AD-A318 987/5INZ).

Stelmack, R. M., Houlihan, M., Doucet, C., & Belisle, M. (1994). Event-related potentials and the detection of deception: A two-stimulus paradigm. *Psychophysiology, 7,* s94.

Tucker, D. M., Liotti, M., Potts, G. F., Russell, G. S., & Posner, M. I. (1994). Spatiotemporal analysis of brain electrical fields. *Human Brain Mapping, 1,* 134-152.

Vendemia, J. M .C., & Buzan, R. F. (2004, April). HD-ERP correlates of workload during deception in two mock crime paradigms. Poster presented at the 11th Annual Cognitive Neuroscience Society (CNS) meeting, San Francisco, CA.

Verleger, R. (1997). On the utility of P3 latency as an index of mental chronometry. *Psychophysiology, 34,* 131-156.

Wilson, G. F., Swain, C. R., & Ullsperger, P. (1998). ERP components elicited in response to warning stimuli: The influence of task difficulty. *Biological Psychology, 47,* 137-158.

# The Boys Totem Town Neurofeedback Project: A Pilot Study of EEG Biofeedback with Incarcerated Juvenile Felons

George Martin, MA
Cynthia L. Johnson, PsyD

**SUMMARY.** Seven male adolescents, ages 14 to 17 who were in a juvenile detention residential treatment program and diagnosed with the combined type of Attention Deficit Hyperactivity Disorder (ADHD-C) or with Conduct Disorder, participated in a study examining the effects of electroencephalographic (EEG) neurofeedback on sustained attention, response inhibition, executive functions, intellectual ability, and memory. All of the participants received 20 sessions of EEG biofeedback therapy in conjunction with treatment received in a residential program.

Pre- and post-treatment measures were collected within one week of treatment, and data were analyzed using an adapted model of Jacobson and Truax's method of clinically significant change (Jacobson & Truax, 1991) which allows criterion scores to be set and 95 percent confidence intervals determined at the level of individual performance on the collected measures. Sixty-four percent experienced improved performance

---

George Martin is a psychologist in private practice in Saint Paul, Minnesota.
Cynthia L. Johnson is a psychologist in private practice in Anoka, Minnesota.
Address correspondence to: George Martin, 127 East County Road C, Little Canada, MN 55117 (E-mail gmartin@usfamily.net).

[Haworth co-indexing entry note]: "The Boys Totem Town Neurofeedback Project: A Pilot Study of EEG Biofeedback with Incarcerated Juvenile Felons." Martin, George, and Cynthia L. Johnson. Co-published simultaneously in *Journal of Neurotherapy* (The Haworth Medical Press, an imprint of The Haworth Press, Inc.) Vol. 9, No. 3, 2005, pp. 71-86; and: *Forensic Applications of QEEG and Neurotherapy* (ed: James R. Evans) The Haworth Medical Press, an imprint of The Haworth Press, Inc., 2005, pp. 71-86. Single or multiple copies of this article are available for a fee from The Haworth Document Delivery Service [1-800-HAWORTH, 9:00 a.m. - 5:00 p.m. (EST). E-mail address: docdelivery@haworthpress.com].

Available online at http://www.haworthpress.com/web/JN
doi:10.1300/J184v09n03_05

after EEG neurofeedback on one or more measures. Clinically significant and reliable improvements were observed on teacher ratings of the Global Executive Composite from the Behavior Rating Inventory of Executive Function (average improvement = .22 mean item raw score points; Gioia, Isquith, Guy, & Kenworthy, 2000). Normal range performance was enhanced on the Composite IQ measure of the Kaufman Brief Intelligence Test (average gain = 9 points; Kaufman & Kaufman, 1990), on the Omissions subscale from the Conners' Continuous Performance Test (average decrease = 13 errors; Conners, 1994) and on the four subtest screening measures from the Wide Range Assessment of Memory and Learning (Sheslow & Adams, 1990), with average gains ranging from 2.0 to 3.67 scaled score points across the four subtests. The results are consistent with previous findings, and suggest that the methodology used for data analysis is a useful tool to assess individual levels of change, and indicate that EEG biofeedback may be a useful adjunct in the treatment of juvenile offenders. *[Article copies available for a fee from The Haworth Document Delivery Service: 1-800-HAWORTH. E-mail address: <docdelivery@haworthpress.com> Website: <http://www.HaworthPress.com>* © 2005 by The Haworth Press, Inc. All rights reserved.]

**KEYWORDS.** Juvenile corrections, neurofeedback, ADHD, adolescents

## INTRODUCTION

Attention Deficit Hyperactivity Disorder (ADHD) is among the most common disorders of childhood, affecting between three and seven percent of the school age population (American Psychiatric Association, 2000). A practical definition of the disorder includes impairment in five areas: impulsivity, inattention, over-arousal, difficulty with gratification, along with emotional lability and external locus of control (Goldstein, 1999). These impaired areas of functioning currently are included in one or more of the three subtypes of the disorder, as defined by the fourth edition of the Diagnostic and Statistical Manual of Mental Disorders-Text Revision (American Psychiatric Association, 2000): predominantly inattentive, predominantly hyperactive-impulsive, and combined types. ADHD and conduct disorders frequently are co-morbid, with a high incidence of both among persons convicted of crimes.

Over the years, numerous studies have been conducted to determine the neurobiological underpinnings of ADHD, with the primary focus being the frontal regions of the brain. There has also been a growing body of research supporting the use of electroencephalographic (EEG) neurofeedback as a primary treatment for ADHD.

## ADHD, Conduct Disorders and the Frontal Regions of the Brain

The frontal lobe theory of ADHD was introduced in the 1930s, when similarities were observed between patients with lesions in the frontal lobe and children with ADHD symptoms (Aman, Roberts, & Pennington, 1998). Both groups were noted to display deficits in response inhibition, inattention, excessive restlessness and distractibility. Since that time, there has been a continuing effort to better understand the functions of the frontal lobe system and how abnormalities in these functions lead to these symptoms.

Other findings of interest regarding frontal lobe function and behavioral disorders in adolescents and children have been found. Of special relevance here are findings regarding brain electrical activity (EEG) in the frontal areas of the cortex. High absolute delta power has been seen in adolescents with oppositional and explosive behaviors (Bauving, Laucht & Schmidt, 2000). Bars, Hevrend, Simpson, and Munger (2001) found atypical frontal brain activation in children diagnosed with oppositional defiant disorder. They noted greater right than left frontal alpha power. A common finding in children with ADHD has been excessive power in slower wave (theta and alpha) portions of the EEG at frontal and central sites, often in combination with abnormally decreased power at higher frequencies.

Since there is evidence that there are deficiencies in attention, impulse control and other executive functions in many persons convicted of crimes, and since these deficiencies are known to be related to brain damage/dysfunction and EEG abnormalities, any treatment with a potential to modify brain function should prove especially useful in correctional settings. The authors conducted an investigation in which incarcerated youths with evidence of problems with attention and impulse control had their residential treatment enhanced with EEG biofeedback (neurofeedback) training designed to help improve regulation of brain function.

## METHOD

This study was conducted using a within subjects, quasi-experimental design, with pre- and post-measures that assessed treatment related change in executive functions. These functions included sustained attention, response inhibition and working memory.

## Participants

The sample included seven male adolescents, ages 14 to 17 years, involved with a correction-based, residential treatment program in Ramsey County, Minnesota. Participants were referred for the EEG treatment if they had a current diagnosis of ADHD, or if a screening completed by the staff psychologist indicated a diagnosis of ADHD or significant problems with impulse control. Table 1 provides information about age and diagnoses of each participant. Individuals with the combined type of ADHD are identified by the abbreviation ADHD-C. Two individuals with a primary diagnosis of Conduct Disorder were included in the sample, due to the high rate of comorbidity with ADHD, and the increased impulsivity individuals with Conduct Disorder display (American Psychiatric Association, 2000).

Participants were briefed about confidentiality and other ethical aspects of participation in this treatment, and signed permission was obtained from parents or legal guardians prior to initiation of the treatment. Participants completed pre- and post-treatment testing, which occurred in a quiet room at the residential facility.

## Measures

*Conners' Continuous Performance Test 3.0* (CPT; Conners, 1994): The CPT is a computer-based measure, where respondents are required to press the computer keyboard space bar when any letter, except the letter "X," appears on the computer monitor. There are 360 trials pre-

TABLE 1. Participant Characteristics

| Client | Age | Primary Diagnosis | Secondary Diagnosis |
|--------|-----|-------------------|---------------------|
| 1 | 16 | Conduct Disorder | None |
| 2 | 15 | Conduct Disorder | None |
| 3 | 17 | ADHD-C | Cannabis Dependence |
| 4 | 15 | ADHD-C | None |
| 5 | 14 | ADHD-C | Major Depression |
| 6 | 15 | ADHD-C | Cannabis Dependence |
| 7 | 17 | ADHD-C | Cannabis Dependence |

sented in 18 consecutive blocks of 20 trials (letter presentations). The 18 blocks are presented with three different inter-stimulus intervals (ISIs). The ISIs are one, two and four seconds, with display times of 250 milliseconds. The order in which the different ISIs are presented varies between blocks. The CPT takes 14 minutes to complete. The scores include 11 measures that reflect attention and impulse control, in addition to an overall index score. These are reported in terms of T-scores and percentiles. The number of omissions (missed targets) an individual makes is the primary measure of sustained attention, while impulsivity is measured by the number of commissions (false hits) made.

*Wide Range Assessment of Memory and Learning* (WRAML; Sheslow & Adams, 1990): This test is designed as a clinical instrument to assess memory and learning functions across the school years. The entire battery consists of nine subtests, yielding three main scales (Verbal Memory Index, Visual Memory Index and Learning Index). These index scores are summed to create a General Memory Index. A Screening Form comprised of four subtests (Picture Memory, Design Memory, Verbal Learning and Story Memory) was used in this study. The correlations between the Screening Form and the complete WRAML standard form are .846 (ages 8 and older) and .864 (ages 9 and older). The Screening Form requires approximately 10 to 15 minutes to complete.

*Behavior Rating of Executive Function* (BRIEF; Gioia, Isquith, Guy & Kenworthy, 2000): This is a rating scale for parents and teachers to complete regarding the executive function-related behaviors of children, ages 5 to 18 years. Both forms contain 86 items, with eight clinical scales assessing the following executive functions: Inhibit, Shift, Emotional Control, Initiate, Working Memory, Plan and Organize Materials, and Monitor. Two validity scales are included which assess inconsistency of responses and negativity. The eight clinical scales are used in computing scores on two broader indexes, Behavioral Regulation and Metacognition. These indexes provide summary information about a child's ability to shift cognitive set and modulate emotions and behavior, along with the ability to cognitively self-manage tasks and monitor performance. The Global Executive Composite is a summary score also derived from the clinical scales.

*Kaufman Brief Intelligence Test* (K-BIT; Kaufman & Kaufman, 1990): This is a brief, individually administered measure of verbal and nonverbal intelligence. It contains two subtests: Vocabulary (including Part A, Expressive Vocabulary and Part B, Definitions), and Matrices. Age-normed standard scores with a mean of 100 and a standard deviation of 15 are provided for the K-Bit IQ Composite score. This composite score has been shown to correlate well with the Wechsler Intelligence Scale for Children-Revised Full Scale IQ score ($r = .8$), supporting the construct validity of the K-Bit IQ Composite score.

## Variables

Variables included: (a) changes in performance on the CPT using the measures of Omissions and Commissions and the overall Index score, (b) changes in scores on the four subtest screening form of the WRAML, (c) changes in teacher ratings on three summary scales of the BRIEF including Behavioral Regulation, Metacognition, and the Global Executive Composite, and (d) changes in the K-BIT Composite score.

## EEG Apparatus

The EEG neurofeedback was provided using a Pentium II laptop computer, a 14-inch active matrix screen and Windows 98, 2nd edition as the operating system. The visual and auditory stimuli for the neurofeedback training were provided using a BrainMaster System Type 2E (BrainMaster Technologies, 2000b) and Brainwave Animation Pro software version 2.00.05 (BrainMaster Technologies, 2000c). The BrainMaster hardware samples at a rate of 120 samples per second, with an input impedance of 10 mega ohms. The amplifier has a bandwidth of .5 to 40 Hz, with a common mode rejection of 90 db.

The Brainwave Animation Pro software filters the EEG data stream into its component bandwidths using third order Butterworth filters, and displays both raw and filtered wave forms on screen. Feedback is provided by means of computer animations that play or pause, and the playing of a single tone. The animations play (progress) and the sound plays when all designated thresholds are being met, playback of the animation and play of the sound pause when the thresholds are not met. A midi tune (user selectable) begins to play after 100 points have been scored within a three-minute period. If the score for any three-minute period is higher than the score for the immediately preceding period a special animation plays.

## Procedure

Seven participants completed both pre- and post-testing using the BRIEF, Conners' CPT, K-BIT and WRAML, and 20 neurofeedback sessions. The pre-testing was completed one week prior to the initiation of neurofeedback training and the post-testing was completed within one week after completion of the training. The training sessions lasted approximately 30 minutes each and occurred two to three times per week. The same training protocol was used with each client. An F3-F4 electrode placement was used with wide band amplitude reduction (2-36Hz), and C3-C4 was used in wide band amplitude reduction (2-30 Hz) and in SMR augmentation (12-15 Hz), coupled with reduction of theta (2-7Hz) and hi-beta (20-36Hz).

Training took place in three 10-minute segments during each training session. The first segment of each session utilized wide band amplitude reduction (2-30Hz) at F3-F4. The second portion included wide band reduction at C3-C4. The third portion included theta (2-7Hz) and high beta (20-36Hz) reduction and SMR (12-15Hz) enhancement at C3-C4. The wideband amplitude reduction thresholds were set so a reward could be given 85% of the time. The SMR protocol thresholds were set so that the total reward percent was approximately 80%.

## Electrode Placement

Electrode placement sites were established using the international 10-20 locations described by Lubar (1995). To place electrodes, the participant's skin surface was cleaned and prepared using NuPrep, a mild abrasive gel. A gold-plated clip electrode prepared with 10-20 Conductive Paste was placed on the ear and used for the ground site. A headband with two, gold-plated electrodes, set in sponges and soaked in saline solution, was used on the active (F3, C3) and reference (F4, C4) sites on the scalp. Proper electrode connections were verified by visually examining the waveform display, as outlined in the BrainMaster General Manuals and Technical Information (BrainMaster Technologies, 2000a, p. U-19). Electrodes with poor connections were removed and the preparation process was repeated.

## Data Collection

During EEG biofeedback training, participants were taken to a room separate from classroom and school activity. Each client was seated in a chair, approximately two feet in front of a laptop computer screen. Each session was conducted in an identical manner across participants. Each session involved the presentation of visual (flying through a landscape scene) and auditory (tone) stimuli that responded to desired changes in EEG, as described above. As each client met the reward criteria, they moved faster through the landscaped scene and heard a pleasant tone to indicate success.

## RESULTS

### Statistical Procedures

The differences obtained between the pre- and post-test scores on the dependent measures provided information about the effectiveness of EEG neurofeedback in modifying the identified executive functions of the participants. Jacobson and Truax's (1991) model of clinically significant change was employed. This model is based on the concept of normative assessment, where an individual client's functioning is compared to that of the normative group employed for that particular assessment instrument. Based on the determination of cut-off scores, one can identify if a client's functioning has improved, deteriorated or remained the same, as a result of the treatment. According to Wiger and Solberg (2001), the additional use of a reliable change index (RCI) serves to determine if the differences between an individual's pre- and post-treatment scores are due to measurement error or the treatment. They outlined the calculation of a RCI, based on a 95% confidence interval, using a formula adapted from Jacobson and Truax's (1991) model. This model is based on the concept of normative assessment, where an individual client's functioning is compared to that of a normative group. Based on the determination of cut-off scores, one can identify if a client's functioning has improved, deteriorated or remained the same, as a result of the treatment. The calculation of a RCI, uses the formula: $RCI = 1.96 \sqrt{2S^2 (1 - r_{tt})}$.

The Z score value of 1.96 represents the 95% confidence interval. The $S$ value is the standard deviation of the scores of the test, and the reliability coefficient is represented by $r_{tt}$. The 95% confidence interval for the RCI is determined by setting cut-off scores that are two standard deviations on either side of the mean of the normative sample scores.

In this study changes in the participants' executive function behaviors, as measured by the BRIEF, Conners' CPT, K-Bit and the screening version of the WRAML, were determined by calculating cut-off scores and RCIs on each test.

### Reliable Change Index/Clinical Significance

Clinically significant change is any change that meets the established confidence level. An RCI was calculated where a minimum number of points of change in the test score was set, based on the reliability coefficient and standard deviation of the test. This established a 95% confidence interval around the cut-off score.

## Results Summary

The results from the data analyses are summarized for the sample in Figures 1 and 2. Figure 2 reflects the total number of participants who showed clinically significant change on each particular measure. Results were viewed in this fashion to illustrate which measures were most sensitive to the changes brought about by neurofeedback.

*Conners' CPT:* The results for one client were not included in the analysis because his performance on the pre-test was invalid. Four individuals decreased the number of omission errors they produced from pre-test to post-test, although only two of these participants scored in the clinical range at pre-test and below this level at post-test. The changes for these latter two participants after EEG neurofeedback reflected a change to normal functioning (RCI = .90). The remaining two individuals' post-test scores indicate normal functioning as well, although they also had performed in the normal range initially (criterion < 17.15). One individual did not show a change in performance, but this must be viewed in light of the fact that he produced no omission errors during either time period. One client produced more omission errors after treatment compared to before treatment, representing clinically significant and reliable deterioration (RCI = .90) although his post-test

FIGURE 1. Results on All Scales

|  | BRI | MC | GEC | CPT Index | Pict Mem | Design Mem | Verbal Learn | Story Mem | Vocab | Matrices | Comp IQ |
|---|---|---|---|---|---|---|---|---|---|---|---|
| #1 | ns | Δ | Δ | 0 | ns | Δ | Δ | Δ | Δ | Δ | Δ |
| #2 | Δ | Δ | Δ | Δ | ns | ns | ns | Δ | Δ | Δ | Δ |
| #3 | Δ | Δ | Δ | invalid | Δ | Δ | ns | Δ | ns | Δ | Δ |
| #4 | Δ | Δ | Δ | ns | ns | ns | ns | Δ | Δ | Δ | Δ |
| #5 | ns | −Δ | −Δ | Δ | Δ | Δ | ns | Δ | ns | ns | Δ |
| #6 | ns | Δ | ns | Δ | Δ | Δ | Δ | ns | ns | ns | Δ |
| #7 | Δ | Δ | ns | Δ | Δ | Δ | Δ | ns | ns | Δ | Δ |

ns = no significant change
−Δ = significant negative change
Δ = significant positive change
0 = pre- and post-test scores were 0

FIGURE 2. Total Changes Per Scale

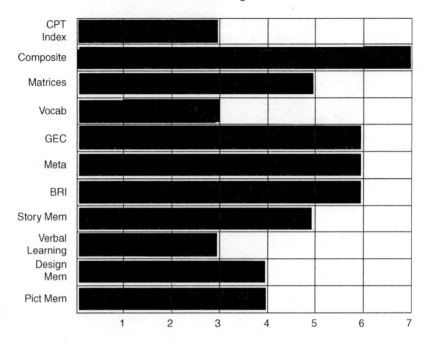

score remained well below the criterion for ADHD. Overall, the participants demonstrated an average decrease of 13 errors from pre-treatment to post-treatment.

The results from the CPT Commissions Scale did not demonstrate reliable change because the standard error of measure (SEM) used to calculate the RCI was quite large (mean SEM = 12.56). As a result, it was difficult for participants to obtain scores outside the band of measurement error (RCI = 14.35).

Five of the seven participants produced usable Conners' CPT Index scores. One produced invalid results, and one achieved a score of 0 on both pre- and post-tests. Of the remaining five, three showed clinically significant positive change, one showed clinically significant negative change and one showed no significant change in either direction. Two of the participants improved their scores from the abnormal to normal range.

*BRIEF:* The Global Executive Composite from the BRIEF, a summary of all changes on that instrument, was believed to provide the best measure of treatment change of the three BRIEF indices analyzed. Four participants scored within the normal range on the Global Executive Composite (RCI = .17) as rated by their teachers, while another individual demonstrated significant change although not achieving a normal result. One client displayed mild deterioration and another failed to show clinically significant change. These results of the BRIEF indicate that five out of seven participants demonstrated a clinically significant and reliable, positive response to the treatment on at least one of the scales.

*WRAML:* Performance on the Verbal Learning subtest was characterized by no change for four participants. The remaining three participants displayed gains averaging 3.67 scaled score points, with one individual improving his performance from below average before treatment to scoring within the normal range after treatment. These results indicate three of the seven participants were able to learn and recall significantly more individual words over a series of trials after treatment, while four participants demonstrated no change.

The Story Memory subtest required participants to listen to a paragraph-length story and repeat it immediately afterward. Four individuals were better able to recall details of the story after treatment, performing in the average range at the time of the post-test (RCI = 1.0). Three of these participants had scored in the average range during the pre-test period; therefore, they improved their already solid abilities. The remaining participant of these four increased his performance from below average prior to treatment to scoring within the normal range after treatment. In addition, another client improved his performance, although he did not reach the criterion level. Finally, two participants did not demonstrate any change on this measure. These results suggest 71% of the sample received a positive benefit in memory for verbal discourse after completion of EEG neurofeedback, averaging 2.0 scaled score points improvement.

Forty-three percent of the sample did not produce meaningful change on the WRAML Picture Memory subtest, a measure of visual memory. Four individuals were able to improve upon their already average range performance after treatment.

The Design Memory subtest of the WRAML provides a measure of visual memory for abstract geometric designs. All participants performed well within the normal range during both measurement periods. Four participants demonstrated clinically significant and reliable improvements in performance (RCI = 1.06), while an additional client was slightly below the RCI cutoff level. The remaining two participants did not produce reliable changes, although one displayed a non-significant trend toward decreased performance after treatment. These results indicate the majority of the sample experienced improved visual memory performance after treatment, with an average increase of 3.5 scaled score points.

*K-BIT:* The Composite IQ measure from the K-Bit provides an estimate of an individual's level of intellectual functioning. Five participants performed within the normal range prior to treatment, and experienced clinically significant and reliable gains in intellectual functioning after treatment (RCI = 2.51). The remaining two participants scored below average on the pre-test results and received scores in the average range after treatment. The gains for all seven participants averaged 9.14 standard score points and ranged from 4 to 18 standard score points. The results indicate that significant improvements in intellectual functioning were consistently observed in the sample.

## DISCUSSION AND CONCLUSION

All of the participants experienced improved performance after EEG neurofeedback on at least one of the dependent variables. Significant gains averaging nine standard score points on the K-BIT IQ Composite were obtained over all seven participants These results are consistent with previous studies, which have reported improved performance on measures of intellectual functioning after neurofeedback (Linden, Habib, & Radojevic, 1996; Lubar, Swartwood, Swartwood, & O'Donnell, 1995; Tansey, 1991). Thompson and Thompson (1998) found an average 12-point gain on the Full Scale IQ index of the Wechsler Intelligence Scales following neurofeedback training.

The teacher ratings on the BRIEF showed consistent improvements across most of the participants. The Global Executive Composite indicated clinically significant improvements for five of seven participants. The improvements reflected gains in aspects of flexible problem-solving, improved regulation of emotional reactions and behavior, and inhibition of inappropriate responses. Six of the participants received scores similar to the instrument's ADHD-C group norm prior to treatment, while only two received such scores after treatment. This suggests that in the residential treatment setting, those participants displayed fewer aggressive behaviors, were able to make better decisions about how to handle problems or conflicts, were able to maintain attention to a greater degree, and had increased awareness of their behaviors after they received EEG neurofeedback.

Results from the WRAML indicated the participants displayed improved performance on various aspects of verbal and nonverbal memory, with five of the individuals who scored in the abnormal range on the pre-test scoring in the normal range on the post-test. In general, all participants improved their scores on at least one subtest of the WRAML, with scores increasing by 1.0 to 7.0 scaled score points. Thus, it seems that neurofeedback training such as that of this study can have positive effects on several types of memory.

Three participants improved their scores on measures from the Conners' CPT and one showed significant decline. The latter's scores, however, were well below the ADHD cutoff level at both assessment periods. Of the four who improved, two had scored at the ADHD level initially. Both of these appeared to respond positively to the neurofeedback, and their scores were at normal levels at post-testing. On average, participants produced 13 fewer CPT Omission errors after treatment, suggesting improved ability to sustain attention.

Overall, the results from the current study demonstrated improved cognitive and executive functioning after EEG neurofeedback. Teacher ratings of the participants' behaviors indicated the most change, and suggest the participants experienced increased behavioral regulation (i.e., they were less impulsive and disruptive). This is an especially important finding inasmuch as problems with behavioral regulation obviously are common in forensic settings.

Changes in CPT performance were not as striking as some of the other measures in the current study. This may have been because Omission errors (reflecting inattention) were not the best measure of the participants' main deficits, and the Commissions subscale from the CPT (reflecting impulsivity) contained too much variability to be useful. It is possible the participants would have experienced greater impairment on other measures of response inhibition, which might have provided more room for improvement after neurofeedback. Given the participants' histories of legal involvement, it is reasonable to assume they demonstrated impulse control problems in everyday life. This is consistent with Barkley's argument that ADHD is primarily a disorder of response inhibition (Barkley, 1997) rather than attention issues. It may have been useful to include reaction time and response variability in the analyses to better explore this possibility.

The mild gains produced in memory and the larger gains in intellectual functioning are interesting (and not necessarily expected), because these areas are not inherently associated with ADHD symptomatology. According to Othmer, Othmer, and Kaiser (1999), however, there is a reasonable explanation for these types of general cognitive improvements that also have been documented by others. These authors suggest the core issue of ADHD "is a disruption or discontinuity in the processes by which different brain regions maintain communication and continuity of mental processing" (p. 299). They note the disruption is global, and not limited to a specific brain region or neurotransmitter system. Because neurofeedback serves to improve the brain's ability to maintain homeostasis and leads to improved stability of the brain's regulatory functions, it may impact brain functioning on a global level and contribute to more efficient cortical communication and processing. Therefore, if neurofeedback influences very basic neurological processes and, as a result, every level of cognitive function is impacted, individuals who perform within normal limits on various IQ measures yet experience significant gains after neurofeedback (as was the case in the current study), may simply be processing information more efficiently. Therefore they are more able to access skills that have developed, but previously were not consistently available.

In the current study, individual levels of improvement or deterioration were assessed using the Reliable Change Index as a measure of clinical significance. This allowed statements to be made regarding the clinical significance and reliability of these changes with 95% confidence. As a result, previous critiques of EEG neurofeedback efficacy research, such as the lack of statistical power, were not relevant for the current study. The use of this methodology demonstrated its sensitivity to neurofeedback treatment-related changes in areas associated with executive and general cognitive functioning. The present findings are consistent with some previous research and suggest that EEG neurofeedback may be a helpful adjunct in the treatment of juvenile offenders. Hopefully this study will serve as a basis for further research in adolescent corrections. Future research using larger samples and control groups should help validate EEG neurofeedback as an effective intervention for adolescent offenders.

## REFERENCES

Aman, C. J., Roberts, R. J., & Pennington, B. F. (1998). A neuropsychological examination of the underlying deficit in attention deficit hyperactivity disorder: Frontal lobe versus right parietal lobe theories. *Developmental Psychology, 34* (5), 956-969.

American Psychiatric Association (2000). *Diagnostic and statistical manual of mental disorders* (4th ed., text revision). Washington, DC: Author.

Barkley, R. A. (1997). *ADHD and the nature of self control.* New York, NY: Guilford Press.

Bars, D., Hevrend, L., Simpson, D., & Munger, J. (2001). Use of visual evoked-potentials studies and EEG data to classify aggressive, explosive behavior of youths. *American Psychiatric Association, 52,* 81-86.

Baving, L., Laucht, L., & Schmidt, M. (2000). Oppositional children differ from healthy children in fronal brain activation. *Journal of Abnormal Child Psychology, 28,* 267-275.

BrainMaster Technologies (2000a). *BrainMaster system type 2E module and BMT software for Windows: General manuals and technical information* [Software manual]. Oakwood Village, OH: Author.

BrainMaster Technologies (2000b). *BrainMaster system type 2E.* Oakwood Village, OH: Author.

BrainMaster Technologies (2000c). *Brainwave animation pro* (Version 2.00.05) [Computer software]. Oakwood Village, OH: Author.

Conners, C. K. (1994). *The Conners' continuous performance test* (Version 3.0). Toronto, Canada: Multihealth Systems.

Gioia, G., Isquith, P., Guy, S., & Kenworthy, L. (2000). *Behavior rating inventory of executive function.* Odessa, FL: Psychological Assessment Resources.

Goldstein, S. (1999). Attention-deficit/hyperactivity disorder. In S. Goldstein & C. R. Reynolds (Eds.), *Handbook of neurodevelopmental and genetic disorders in children* (pp. 154-184). New York, NY: Guilford Press.

Jacobson, N. S., & Truax, P. (1991). Clinical significance: A statistical approach to defining meaningful change in psychotherapy research. *Journal of Consulting and Clinical Psychology, 59,* 12-19.

Kaufman, A., & Kaufman, N. (1990). *Kaufman brief intelligence test.* Circle Pines, MN: American Guidance Service.

Linden, M., Habib, T., & Radojevic, V. (1996). A controlled study of EEG biofeedback effects on cognitive and behavioral measures with attention-deficit and learning disabled children. *Biofeedback and Self Regulation, 21,* 35-49.

Lubar, J. F. (1995). Neurofeedback for the management of attention deficit/hyperactivity disorder. In M. Schwartz (Ed.), *Biofeedback* (pp. 493-522). New York: Guilford.

Lubar, J. F., Swartwood, M. O., Swartwood, J. N., & O'Donnell, P. H. (1995). Evaluation of the effectiveness of EEG neurofeedback training for ADHD in a clinical setting as measured by changes in T.O.V.A. scores, behavioral ratings and WISC-R performance. *Biofeedback and Self Regulation, 20,* 83-99.

Othmer, S., Othmer, S., & Kaiser, D. (1999). EEG biofeedback: An emerging model for its global efficacy. In J. Evans & A. Abarnel (Eds.), *Introduction to quantitative EEG and neurofeedback* (pp. 244-310). San Diego, CA: Academic Press.

Sheslow, D., & Adams, W. (1990). *Wide range assessment of memory and learning.* Wilmington, DE: Jastak Associates.

Tansey, M. (1991). Wechsler (WISC-R) changes following treatment of learning disabilities via EEG neurofeedback training in a private practice setting. *Australian Journal of Psychology, 43,* 147-153.

Thompson, L., & Thompson, M. (1998). Neurofeedback combined with training in metacognitive strategies: Effectiveness in students with ADD. *Applied Psychophysiology and Biofeedback, 23* (4), 243-263.

Wiger, D., & Solberg, K. (2001). *Tracking mental health outcomes: A therapist's guide to measuring client progress, analyzing data and improving your practice.* New York: John Wiley and Sons.

# Neurofeedback with Juvenile Offenders: A Pilot Study in the Use of QEEG-Based and Analog-Based Remedial Neurofeedback Training

Peter N. Smith, PsyD
Marvin W. Sams, ND

**SUMMARY.** *Introduction.* Atypical EEG and neuropsychological indicators have been observed among offenders. Dangerous offenders treated with a combined program that included neurofeedback (EEG biofeedback) and galvanic skin response (GSR) biofeedback demonstrated reduction in recidivism (Quirk, 1995). This study was designed to further evaluate the EEG findings of youth offenders and to provide an initial report on the effectiveness of a task-oriented analog/QEEG-based remedial neurofeedback training approach.

*Method.* Five offenders with significant psychopathology were referred for treatment. The group was evaluated with attentional testing and analog/QEEG assessment prior to and following neurotherapy. Treatment consisted of 20 or 40 sessions of a task-activated analog/ QEEG-based approach. Another group of thirteen offenders were as-

---

Peter N. Smith is in independent practice in Tucson, Arizona.

Marvin W. Sams is Director of The Sams Center for Optimal Performance, Dallas, Texas.

Address correspondence to: Peter N. Smith, 11300 East Broadway Boulevard, Tucson, AZ 85748 (E-mail: pns001@aol.com).

[Haworth co-indexing entry note]: "Neurofeedback with Juvenile Offenders: A Pilot Study in the Use of QEEG-Based and Analog-Based Remedial Neurofeedback Training." Smith, Peter N., and Marvin W. Sams. Co-published simultaneously in *Journal of Neurotherapy* (The Haworth Medical Press, an imprint of The Haworth Press, Inc.) Vol. 9, No. 3, 2005, pp. 87-99; and: *Forensic Applications of QEEG and Neurotherapy* (ed: James R. Evans) The Haworth Medical Press, an imprint of The Haworth Press, Inc., 2005, pp. 87-99. Single or multiple copies of this article are available for a fee from The Haworth Document Delivery Service [1-800-HAWORTH, 9:00 a.m. - 5:00 p.m. (EST). E-mail address: docdelivery@haworthpress.com].

Available online at http://www.haworthpress.com/web/JN
doi:10.1300/J184v09n03_06

sessed with attentional testing and provided with neurotherapy following QEEG assessment.

*Results.* For all of the youth trained, in the analog/QEEG group, pre-
vs. post-audio and visual attention testing demonstrated significant improvement within 20 remedial sessions. Three of the five youth showed
rapid advancement in a residential grading system. Staff observational
ratings suggested behavioral improvement in the QEEG group who in
general were in training for a longer period of time.

*Conclusion.* EEG abnormalities and deficits in neuropsychological
testing were found among offenders. Neurotherapy as an adjunctive treatment appears to hold promise for improvement in cognitive performance
as well as recidivism. It is anticipated that different neurofeedback protocols may enhance outcomes. *[Article copies available for a fee from The
Haworth Document Delivery Service: 1-800-HAWORTH. E-mail address:
<docdelivery@haworthpress.com> Website: <http://www.HaworthPress.com>
© 2005 by The Haworth Press, Inc. All rights reserved.]*

**KEYWORDS.** Juvenile offenders, prison, neurotherapy, neurofeedback, QEEG-based neurofeedback, analog-based neurofeedback, remedial neurofeedback training

## INTRODUCTION

Quirk (1995) demonstrated a reduction in recidivism in an adult offender population with a combined protocol of neurofeedback (EEG
biofeedback) and galvanic skin response (GSR) training. While Quirk's
work focused on adults, another clinician studied the effects of neurofeedback on incarcerated adolescent felons (Martin, 2002). This younger population also demonstrated benefit from neurofeedback intervention, with enhanced learning capacity and improved behavior.

The benefit of neurofeedback in remediating problems with attention, performance, and behavior is well known. It is therefore surprising
that studies with offenders have been so slow in coming. The positive
outcomes in the Quirk and Martin studies, combined with the need to
address known psychological and neurological issues of those in the
prison population, suggest a more extensive evaluation of neurofeedback should be undertaken.

The purpose of this study is to expand the current research in the use
of neurofeedback in those convicted of criminal activity, with emphasis

on the juvenile population. The authors also compared traditional neuro-feedback protocols with techniques developed by the co-author.

## Basis of Study

Juvenile offenders are often compromised neurologically. For example, Attention Deficit Hyperactivity Disorder (ADHD), addictive disorders, and impaired neuropsychological functioning are known to be widespread in the offender population. Hyperactive youth, especially those exhibiting antisocial behaviors, are at significant risk for criminal behavior (Satterfield & Schell, 1997; Mannuzza & Klein, 2000). As neurofeedback has demonstrated the ability to reduce hyperkinesis and impulsivity in those with ADHD (e.g., Lubar & Shouse, 1976, 1977; Shouse & Lubar, 1979; Lubar, Swartwood, Swartwood, & O'Donnell, 1995; Lubar, 2003; Tansey & Bruner, 1983; Tansey, 1993), the question follows: Would decreasing hyperactivity and impulsivity in the criminal population reduce recidivism? Additionally, since the younger the subject at first arrest, the greater the likelihood of chronic and accelerating offenses, would neurofeedback deter future criminal activity in youthful offenders?

Research demonstrating the effectiveness of neurofeedback in addictive disorders includes the work of Peniston and Kulkosky (1989, 1991) and Saxby and Peniston (1995). While the authors know of few studies specifically evaluating the possible benefit of neurofeedback in addicted youth offenders, many in the juvenile corrections population have addictions and therefore should be good candidates for such intervention.

Studies in men convicted of violent crimes have found abnormal electroencephalographic (EEG) activity and impaired neuropsychological functioning. In one study (Evans & Park, 1997) indications of frontal and right hemisphere dysfunction were found in 20 men convicted of murder. Abnormalities noted were those associated with coherence, phase and amplitude asymmetries using an EEG normative reference database. In a study with a similar population (Evans & Claycomb, 1999), the presence of paroxysmal delta waves (primarily right lateral frontal) and/or excessive relative power in alpha frequencies at frontal or lateral frontal sites was associated with a history of dissociative experiences or out-of-character behavior that sometimes involved violence. In still another quantitative EEG (QEEG) study, reduced EEG comodulation was found in a sample of death penalty cases which, according to the author, suggests brain dysfunction (Weinstein, 2002). Other research confirms that neuropsychological brain dysfunction and structural irregularities in the prefrontal cortex are highly correlated with violence and psychopathic behaviors (Raine, 1993).

Overwhelming evidence that cerebral dysfunction can produce disturbed, often criminal behavior is offered in a treatise by Flor-Henry (1983). Temporal lobe epilepsy, in particular, can produce psychic aberrations, fugue states, and unusual behavior. Traumatic brain injury is associated with memory difficulties, problems with attention and concentration, lassitude, disturbance of sleep, irritability, depression, and headache (Kwentis, Hart, Peck, & Kornstein, 1985; Gennarelli, 1986; Prigatano & Pepping, 1987).

Many clinicians utilize neurofeedback training to remediate such neurological and clinical issues. For example, alleviating the symptoms of head injury (see Hoffman, Stockdale, & Van Egren, 1996), reducing seizure activity (a sequela of brain injury and other major types of genetic and acquired brain disease; Sterman & Friar,1972; Sterman, 2000), and learning disabilities (Thornton & Carmody, 2005; Tansey, 1993).

### Study Objectives

The present study investigates whether certain specific neurofeedback interventions impact neurological and behavioral measures in adolescent offenders. In a previously reported study performed with an eating disordered population (Sams & Smith, 2004), the authors compared clinical outcomes with three different approaches to neurofeedback training: symptom-based, quantitative EEG-based, and a combined analog and quantitative EEG-based training that included task-activated neurofeedback protocols, heart rate variability biofeedback, and cortical blood flow training. The present investigation was designed to further evaluate outcomes with two of those three previously used neurofeedback methods–the quantitative EEG-based and analog/quantitative EEG-based approaches. Since Quirk (1995) reported that increasing the number of sessions enhances outcome effectiveness, we also sought to test this.

## METHODS

### Group One

*Participants.* Thirteen incarcerated youthful offenders were referred for neurofeedback training to a program carried out by trained correctional staff and supervised by the first author, a licensed clinical psychologist with training and experience in neurotherapy. The group ranged from 13 to 17 years of age. All participants had a history of multiple criminal offenses and drug abuse/dependence. Some had committed actual crimes while under the influence of drugs. The group consisted of eleven males and two females, with the predominant ethnicity being Hispanic (11 Hispanics vs. 2 Caucasians). The majority of male subjects had a background of mixed substance abuse, while the females were self-reported as addicted to methamphetamines. No information was available regarding socio-economic status.

*Procedure.* Each participant and/or guardian reviewed and signed informed consent forms and received both a written and verbal overview of the training process. The correctional staff completed weekly behavioral forms rating cooperation and completion of assignments and chores on 8 of the 13 subjects. (Five participants were housed at a facility that used a different rating system so their ratings were not considered in data analysis.) In the rating system, youth progress from the lowest level (one) in half steps depending upon cooperative behavior (no adverse behavioral incidents, and completion of chores and assignments) to the top level of seven. A minimum score of five must be achieved before the youth is eligible to be discharged from the facility, a seven being even more desirable.

A TOVA continuous performance test (Greenburg & Waldman, 1993) that evaluates visual attention was administered before training commenced and after session 20. An appropriately sized ECI Electrode-Cap (Electrode-Cap International, Eaton, OH) was placed on the participant's head, and adjusted for symmetry and proper electrode placement. The electrodes were filled with conductive gel using a blunted needle, and impedances reduced to 5 K ohms or below by gently abrading the scalp at the electrode site. EEG data were recorded with a Lexicor 24-channel digital EEG recording device using Neurolex™ software. Two conditions, eyes-open and eyes-closed, were recorded for approximately five minutes each. A sampling rate of 128 samples per second was used, with the high pass filter in the off position.

The recorded data were transferred to Lexicor Medical Technology, Inc., Boulder, CO via e-mail attachment for interpretation and training recommendations. Training protocol selection was based on statistical deviations from a proprietary database (DataLex™). Priority was assigned to adjusting inappropriate amplitudes, followed by asymmetry, coherence, and phase training. Training recommendations were specific for the eyes-open and eyes-closed conditions.

Training sessions were conducted by trained correctional staff supervised by a licensed psychologist certified in biofeedback. All training sessions were done on Lexicor equipment using Biolex™ software. Electrode impedances were reduced to 10 K ohms or less for all biofeedback sessions. Participants were allowed to choose displays for visual feedback and to adjust audio controls to a comfortable level. Adjustments were made to baseline threshold settings after a two-minute baseline recording. Individual training session times ranged from 30 to 40 minutes, depending on the specified protocol. EEG data were collected at the end of each training session.

## Group Two

*Participants.* Five male juvenile offenders were referred for neurofeedback training. The group ranged in age from 13 to 17 years. All had multiple arrests (range of three to nine). Three of the five had gang affiliation, and four had backgrounds of substance abuse or dependence. Two had criminal offenses connected to sexual exploitation and assault. The participant with no substance abuse history had symptoms of ADHD and multiple arrests for larceny. Ethnic background was mixed, with three participants of Hispanic origin, one Caucasian and one African-American. Four had been incarcerated previously. One participant from Group One was later transferred to Group Two. He received ten treatment sessions according to Group Two procedures, after receiving 24 sessions using methods as described for Group One.

*Procedure.* As in Group One, each participant and/or guardian signed consent forms and received both a written and verbal overview of the training process. An IVA Continuous Performance Test (BrainTrain, Inc., Richmond, VA), a test of ability to sustain auditory and visual response control and attention over a 15-minute period (Sandford, 1995; Seckler, Burns, Montgomery, & Sandford, 1995), was administered before neurofeedback training.

For the initial EEG data collection, an appropriate sized ECI Electrode-Cap was placed symmetrically on the head; the electrodes cavities were filled with electrode gel and impedances reduced to 5 K ohms or less by gently abrading the scalp with a blunted needle.

As in Group One, a Lexicor 24-channel digital EEG recording device with NeuroLex™ software was used to collect data. A sampling rate of 128 samples per second, with the high pass filter off, was used for three conditions: eyes-open, eyes-closed, and task activation. The task activation process required the playing of Tetris, a visual-spatial video game, on a Game Boy, a hand-held video game system. The analog EEG data for the three conditions were visually analyzed for disturbances in background activity and to determine if transient focal, asymmetric, epileptiform, or inappropriate generalized activity were present. All data were reformatted to include at least one sequential (scalp-to-scalp recording) montage to visually enhance possible transient focal data. The EEG was then visually edited for artifacts, and all possible artifacts deleted prior to statistical analysis. EEG and QEEG analysis and training recommendations were provided using clinical strategies created around neurological inefficiencies.

Training priority was given to the inefficiencies found in the analog EEG patterning (for example, unstable background activity, paroxysmal activity, significant asymmetries, focal slow waves, spike activity). Next, priority was assigned to inefficient cortical circuits, specifically, coherence and phase deviations found in a lifespan normative reference database (NeuroRep).

Each participant wore an appropriately sized ECI Electrode-Cap for training. A minimum of eleven electrodes (Cz, Fp1, Fp2, F3, F4, P3, P4, F7, F8, T3, T4, and ground) were filled with electrode gel. Other electrode sites were filled as necessary for the specific training protocol. Impedances were reduced to 5 K ohms or less before the baseline data were collected.

A baseline condition preceded all neurofeedback sessions to compare current with previous sessions. An 11-channel, task activated (playing Tetris on Game Boy) baseline was recorded in Neurolex™, using a sampling rate of 128, for a minimum of 80 (two second) epochs. No audio tones were used during the baseline condition.

After the no-audio baseline recording, the trainer adjusted the volume of headphones and placed the headphone pads comfortably over the participant's ears. The participant continued playing the video game as high-pitched tones provided the audio-based neurofeedback training information.

Each session consisted of two or three five-minute, synergistically compatible training protocols (as determined from research by the co-author with other persons with a variety of neurological and psychological symptoms). The training segments were always at the same electrode site(s), using a specific scalp electrode to a combined ear reference linkage, a sequential ("bipolar," or scalp-to-scalp) montage, or a Linear Channel Combination (LLC) montage incorporating the sum of four to seven electrode sites. Each five-minute protocol was a different training band, utilizing a group of frequencies in the 0.5 to 120 Hz range.

The training protocols selected were those shown to decrease delta (0.5-3 Hz), theta (3-6 Hz), alpha_a (8-10 Hz) and/or alpha_f (8-12 Hz), while increasing 13Hz (11.5-14.5 Hz), alpha_b (10-12 Hz), beta1 (15-20 Hz), and/or beta2 (20-28 Hz). These were protocols that had clinically demonstrated the ability to stabilize ongoing background activity (reduce paroxysmal activity and unstable patterning), and remediate inefficiencies found in normative EEG reference database reports. These included: Increase magnitude difference between a pair of scalp electrodes or a scalp to combined ear reference; decrease magnitude difference between two scalp electrodes or a scalp to combined ear reference; increase or decrease synchrony (synchrony defined as 50% coherence and 50% phase) between two scalp sites or multi-electrode sites simultaneously; decrease peak amplitude + synchrony (a mathematical expression of first selecting the peak amplitude of a frequency band, then decreasing the synchrony between two or several electrodes sites simultaneously); appropriate coherence and phase training [the "opposite" of the deviation(s) reported on an age appropriate normative EEG reference database] between electrode pairs shown on the database report, or more diffusely, using multi-site training (if larger areas of deviations are found). Neurofeedback reinforcement was provided by magnitude regulated, high pitched tones (created by the trainer adjusting the y-axis for maximum high pitch) as the subject processed and responded to the complex task (playing Tetris).

Immediately following each neurofeedback training session, the subject completed five minutes of heart rate variability training (Heart Math, Boulder Creek, CA) using diaphragmatic breathing techniques with visual feedback only. This, in turn, was followed by five minutes of frontal (mid-forehead placement) cortical blood flow training (Bio-Comp Research, Los Angeles, CA) under task (playing Tetris) with auditory feedback.

Each participant received either 20 or 40 training sessions as described. The youth who transferred into Group Two from Group One received 10 additional training sessions according to Group Two methods. The IVA visual-auditory continuous performance testing was repeated near the time of the last session and compared to the pre-training data. Pre- and post-EEG data were collected and compared, including an analysis using the Excel statistical program to compare magnitude changes in eight frequency bands at 19 electrode sites. A weekly log and behavioral rating scores were kept by the staff on each participant as described for Group One.

## RESULTS

Pre- to post-training scores were compared. Paired sample T-tests were performed to assess changes in pre- and post-training scores from the TOVA and IVA tests, and from behavioral rating scales as applicable for each group. Scores based on invalid test administration and other invalid scores were dropped from the comparisons, so the total sample size was reduced in Group One from 13 to 8 and one of the 8 subjects provided little valid TOVA data. Results are shown in Tables 1 and 2.

The only significant difference for Group One was change in behavior level from pre-training (mean = 2.9) to session 20 (mean = 6.7). Behavior Level ratings performed by staff range from 1 (least cooperative) to 7 (most cooperative). For Group Two significant differences were found for Auditory Attention Quotients (AAQ) and Visual Attention Quotients (VAQ). The difference was nearly significant for Visual Response Control Quotient (VRCQ) and not significant for the Auditory Response Control Quotient (ARCQ).

Post-training status of Group Two members was followed for a period of six months. Three of the original five participants received 34 or 40 treatment sessions, and successfully completed probation with no arrests. Two of the five received 20 training sessions. While these two offenders showed improvement on attention-related cognitive tests, behavioral ratings did not improve. As a result, probation was not com-

TABLE 1. TOVA and Behavioral Scores, Pre-Training vs. Post-Session 20 for Group One.

|  | Pre-Training | Post-Training | p value |
|---|---|---|---|
| Omission errors | 107.3 | 94.7 | .219 |
| Commission errors | 105.1 | 107.1 | .506 |
| Response time | 111.3 | 106.7 | .557 |
| RT Variability | 103.3 | 102.3 | .928 |
| Post-Commission errors | 5.8 | 4.9 | .474 |
| Behavioral levels | 2.9 | 6.7 | .003* |

*indicates significant difference

TABLE 2. IVA and Behavior Scores Pre-Training vs. Post-Session 20 for Group Two.

|  | Pre-Training | Post-Training | p value |
|---|---|---|---|
| ARCQ | 75.0 | 85.4 | .123 |
| VRCQ | 76.8 | 94.8 | .051 |
| AAQ | 79.6 | 96.2 | .049* |
| VAQ | 74.2 | 91.2 | .043* |
| Hyper-activity | 7.4 | 2.8 | .172 |
| Behavioral level | 1.2 | 2.8 | .099 |

*indicates significant difference

pleted within the six months of the study. There was no opportunity to follow the outcome of Group One participants after cessation of training.

## DISCUSSION

This investigation has a number of shortcomings. The small number of subjects in each group severely restricted statistical treatment of the pre/post training and group comparisons. The lack of matched control groups, the variable training times both within and across groups, and the failure to control for large differences in pre-training test and behavioral rating scores among participants are factors that need to be considered in future research of this type. Furthermore, factors such as determining whether observed behavioral and cognitive changes are causally related to neurofeedback training alone, to a combination with other concurrent treatment, or to other behavioral modification training within participants' institutional settings must be considered. The provision of more extensive and detailed information on the long-term social/psychological adjustment of participants is also a missing factor and should be considered in future research.

These shortcomings considered, neurofeedback training did seem to show favorable impact on cognitive functioning and behavior in these two groups of juvenile offenders. This investigation of two neurofeedback training approaches for juvenile offenders suggests different outcomes that appear to depend on the methods employed. Group One training was based on QEEG results, whereas Group Two training

(a) used protocols that addressed patterns found in both the analog EEG and QEEG analysis, (b) used protocols shown to reduce slow activity (below 10 Hz) and increase fast activity (above 10 Hz) or to reduce magnitude globally at all electrode sites, (c) trained during a task-activation condition, and (d) supplemented neurofeedback training with heart rate variability biofeedback and cortical blood flow training.

Findings of this pilot study provide some suggestions to guide future research. First, there is some evidence that the combined analog and QEEG-based training protocols of Group Two may be more effective for facilitating cognitive changes (decreases in impulsiveness and improvement in sustained attention) than protocols based on QEEG data alone. Giving further weight to the analog/QEEG-based approach are the similar results the authors found in an eating disordered population (Sams & Smith, 2004).

Secondly, there was support for earlier findings that more training sessions lead to greater improvement in behavior, and thus potentially less recidivism. Quirk (1995) observed that effectiveness of neurofeedback with incarcerated persons increased as a function of the number of training sessions done. At least as far as behavioral ratings are concerned, the data from both groups of the present study lend support to this idea. Group One participants (21-57 sessions) who had behavioral rating data available showed ratings improvement over the course of treatment and the three participants in Group Two who had more than 20 sessions improved while the two who had 20 sessions did not.

Group One participants' training extended over an average of 20.6 weeks versus just 7.6 weeks for participants of Group Two. It is not known if the lower behavioral ratings for the two Group Two participants with only 20 sessions were more a function of number of sessions or of time. Follow up was not possible to help determine which was more likely. These issues of combined analog and QEEG-based training as superior, and number of sessions versus duration of training should be addressed in greater depth by future research.

Several studies have shown that a high percentage of incarcerated persons suffer from brain damage or dysfunction, with related problems in behavioral control, attention, and learning. This clinical research study and growing numbers of research results and clinical reports suggest that neurofeedback is useful in facilitating recovery from many such conditions (Walker, 2004). For the benefit of those at high risk to commit crimes, and of their potential victims in society, there is a pressing need for well-designed research studies to explore the use of neurofeedback (and other biofeedback procedures) with both adult and juvenile offenders. Hopefully, the present study will encourage others to explore the possible benefit of neurofeedback in preventing recidivism and rehabilitating some of society's most troubled individuals.

## REFERENCES

Evans, J., & Claycomb, S. (1999). Abnormal QEEG patterns associated with dissociation and violence. *Journal of Neurotherapy, 3* (2), 21-27.
Evans, J., & Park, N. (1997). Quantitative EEG findings among men convicted of murder. *Journal of Neurotherapy, 2* (2), 31-39.
Flor-Henry, P. (1983). *Cerebral basis of psychopathology.* Littleton, MA: John Wright–PSG Inc.
Gennarelli, T. A. (1986). Mechanisms and pathophysiology of cerebral concussion. *Journal of Head Trauma Rehabilitation, 1,* 23-30.
Greenberg, L. M., & Waldman, I. D. (1993). Developmental normative data on the test of variables of attention (TOVA®). *Journal of Child and Adolescent Psychiatry, 34* (6), 1019-1030.
Hoffman, D. A., Stockdale, S., & Van Egren, L. (1996). EEG neurofeedback in the treatment of mild traumatic brain injury [Abstract]. *Clinical Electroencephalography, 27* (2), 6.
Kwentis, J. A., Hart, R. P., Peck, E. T., & Kornstein, S. (1985). Psychiatric implication of closed head trauma. *Psychosomatics, 26,* 8-15.
Lubar, J. F. (2003). Neurofeedback for the management of attention deficit/hyperactivity disorders. Chapter in M. S. Schwartz & F. Andrasik (Eds.), *Biofeedback: A practitioner's guide* (3rd ed., pp. 409-437). New York: Guilford.
Lubar, J. F., & Shouse, M. N. (1976). EEG behavioral changes in a hyperactive child concurrent training of the sensorimotor rhythm (SMR): A preliminary report. *Biofeedback and Self Regulation, 9* (1), 1-23.
Lubar, J. F., & Shouse, M. N. (1977). Use of biofeedback in the treatment of seizure disorders and hyperactivity. *Advances in Clinical Child Psychology, 1,* 204-251.
Lubar, J. F., Swartwood, M. O., Swartwood, J. N., & O'Donnell, P. H. (1995). Evaluation of the effectiveness of EEG neurofeedback training for ADHD in a clinical setting as measured by changes in TOVA scores, behavioral ratings, and WISC-R performance. *Biofeedback and Self-Regulation, 20* (1), 83-99.
Mannuzza, S., & Klein, R. G. (2000). Long-term prognosis in attention deficit/hyperactivity disorder. *Child and Adolescent Psychiatric Clinics of North America, 9,* 711-726.
Martin, G. (2002, September). EEG biofeedback with incarcerated adolescent felons. Paper presented at International Society for Neuronal Regulation Annual Conference, Scottsdale, AZ.
Peniston, E. G., & Kulkosky, P. J. (1989). Alpha-theta brainwave training and beta-endorphin levels in alcoholics. *Alcohol: Clinical and Experimental Research, 13* (2), 271-279.
Peniston, E. G., & Kulkosky, P. J. (1991). Alcoholic personality and alpha-theta brainwave training. *Medical Psychotherapy, 2,* 37-55.

Prigatano, G. P., & Pepping, M. (1987). Neuropsychological status before and after mild head injury: A case report. *Barrow Neurological Institute Quarterly, 3*, 18-21.

Quirk, D. A. (1995). Composite biofeedback conditioning and dangerous offenders: III. *Journal of Neurotherapy. 1* (2), 44-54.

Raine, A. (1993). *The psychopathology of crime: Criminal behavior as a clinical disorder.* Orlando, FL: Academic Press.

Sams, M. W., & Smith, P. (2004, August). The neurological basis of eating disorders II. Follow-up report of adding symptom-based, QEEG-based and analog/QEEG-based remedial neurofeedback training to traditional eating disorders treatment plans. Paper presented at International Society for Neuronal Regulation Annual Conference, Ft. Lauderdale, FL.

Sandford, J. (1995, August). Validity of the IVA integrated visual and auditory continuous performance test. Paper presented at American Psychological Association Annual Conference, New York, NY.

Satterfield, J., & Schell, A. (1997). A prospective study of hyperactive boys with conduct problems and normal boys: Adolescent and adult criminality. *Journal of the American Academy of Child and Adolescent Psychiatry, 36* (12), 1726-1735.

Saxby, E., & Peniston, E. G. (1995). Alpha-theta brainwave neurofeedback training: An effective treatment for male and female alcoholics with depressive symptoms. *Journal of Clinical Psychology, 51* (5), 685-693.

Seckler, P., Burns W., Montgomery D., & Sandford, J. (1995, October). A reliability study of IVA: Integrated visual and auditory continuous performance test. Paper presented at CHADD, Washington, DC.

Shouse, M. N., & Lubar, J. F. (1979). Sensorimotor rhythm (SMR) operant conditioning and methylphenidate in the treatment of hyperkinesis. *Biofeedback and Self-Regulation, 4,* 299-311.

Sterman, M. B. (2000). Basic concepts and clinical findings in the treatment of seizure disorders with EEG operant conditioning. *Clinical Electroencephalography, 31* (1), 45-55.

Sterman, M. B., & Friar, L. (1972). Suppression of seizures in epileptics following sensorimotor EEG feedback training. *Electroencephalography and Clinical Neurophysiology, 33,* 89-95.

Tansey, M. A. (1993). Ten year stability of EEG biofeedback results for a hyperactive boy who failed fourth grade perceptually impaired class. *Biofeedback and Self Regulation, 18* (1), 33-34.

Tansey, M. A., & Bruner, R. L. (1983). EMG and EEG biofeedback training in the treatment of a 10-year-old boy with a developmental reading disorder. *Biofeedback and Self Regulation, 8,* 25-37.

Thornton, K. E., & Carmody, D. P. (2005). Electroencephalogram biofeedback for reading disability and traumatic brain injury. *Child and Adolescent Psychiatric Clinics of North America, 14* (1), 137-162.

Walker, J. (2004). A neurologist's advice for mental health professionals on the use of QEEG and neurofeedback. *Journal of Neurotherapy, 8* (2), 97-103.

Weinstein, R. (2002, September). QEEG in death penalty evaluations. Paper presented at International Society for Neuronal Regulation Annual Conference, Scottsdale, AZ.

# School Shootings, High School Size, and Neurobiological Considerations

## David A. Kaiser, PhD

**SUMMARY.** In the last decade 17 multiple-injury student school shootings have occurred in the United States, 13 at high schools and 4 at middle schools. Research suggests that high schools function best academically as well as socially at enrollments around 600 (150 students per grade), the natural group size of humans. Eleven of 13 high school shootings occurred in schools with enrollments over 600 students, and many with over 1,000 students. Violent and antisocial behavior is associated with deficits in social information processing, which is necessarily exacerbated by complex social environments. School shootings may be in part a response to the unprecedented social complexity of large schools. Median public high school enrollment now stands at 1,200 in suburbs and 1,600 in cities despite the fact that smaller schools are superior to large schools on nearly all academic and social measures of success including graduation rate, student satisfaction, conduct infractions, athletic participation, absenteeism, and dropout rate. Educational institutions should adapt to the neurobiological limitations of children instead

David A. Kaiser is Co-Editor of the *Journal of Neurotherapy* and affiliated with the Rochester Institute of Technology, Rochester, New York.

Address correspondence to: David A. Kaiser, P.O. Box 374, Churchville, NY 14428 (E-mail: davidkaiser@yahoo.com).

[Haworth co-indexing entry note]: "School Shootings, High School Size, and Neurobiological Considerations." Kaiser, David A. Co-published simultaneously in *Journal of Neurotherapy* (The Haworth Medical Press, an imprint of The Haworth Press, Inc.) Vol. 9, No. 3, 2005, pp. 101-115; and: *Forensic Applications of QEEG and Neurotherapy* (ed: James R. Evans) The Haworth Medical Press, an imprint of The Haworth Press, Inc., 2005, pp. 101-115. Single or multiple copies of this article are available for a fee from The Haworth Document Delivery Service [1-800-HAWORTH, 9:00 a.m. - 5:00 p.m. (EST). E-mail address: docdelivery@haworthpress.com].

of forcing children to adapt to the unnatural requirements of such institutions. *[Article copies available for a fee from The Haworth Document Delivery Service: 1-800-HAWORTH. E-mail address: <docdelivery@haworthpress.com> Website: <http://www.HaworthPress.com> © 2005 by The Haworth Press, Inc. All rights reserved.]*

**KEYWORDS.** High school size, natural group size, social intelligence, school violence, school shootings

## INTRODUCTION

From 1970 to 1993 the homicide rate for teenagers 15 to 19 years of age increased nearly three-fold while it declined for adults 30 years and older (Stanton, Baldwin, & Rachuba, 1997). Between 1992 and 2001, 323 school-associated violent deaths occurred in the United States (Stephens, 2003). In the past decade we have witnessed a very disturbing form of adolescent violence, the mass random shooting of students by other students in public schools. Since 1996, 17 multiple-injury student school shootings occurred in the United States which took the lives of 39 children and 13 adults, and injured 111.

Social-related neurocognitive deficits may predispose many individuals to aggression and violence (Dodge, Pettit, McClaskey, & Brown, 1986; Bradshaw & Garbarino, 2004; Silver, Goodman, Knoll, Isakov, & Modai, 2005). The right ventromedial prefrontal cortex, as well as other areas of the right hemisphere and prefrontal cortex, mediate much of social cognition, individuation of others, and social conduct (Tranel, Bechara, & Denburg, 2002; Mason & Macrae, 2004; Mosch, Max, & Tranel, 2005). Acquired sociopathy, for example, is associated with damage to right orbitofrontal cortex (Blair & Cipolotti, 2000) and socially undesirable behavior is more commonly associated with right-sided than left-sided frontotemporal dementia (Mychack, Kramer, Boone, & Miller, 2001; Mendez, Chen, Shapira, & Miller, 2005). Neuroimaging investigations also report abnormal prefrontal circuitry and activity to be associated with violence and antisociality, especially on the right side (Sterzer, Stadler, Krebs, Kleinschmidt, & Poustka, 2005; Bassarath, 2001; Evans & Claycomb, 1999; Evans & Park, 1997; Deckel, Hesselbrock, & Bauer, 1996). Quantitative EEG studies of violent men find either evidence of right hemisphere dysfunction (Evans & Park, 1997) or greater left-sided activation (Convit, Czobor, & Volavka,

1991; Deckel et al., 1996), which is consistent with right hemisphere dysfunction. Evans and Park (1997) also reported more anterior than posterior QEEG abnormalities in a sample of death row inmates.

However, brain damage or dysfunctions are obviously not the only factors behind violent behavior in school-aged persons. All adolescent primates strive for social status, especially males. The use of aggression, even violence, to improve one's social status is nothing new to our species or order (Wrangham & Wilson, 2004). Decades of research link aggression to social status in humans and nonhuman animals. Low peer acceptance is associated with aggression and conduct problems in children (Newcomb, Bukowski, & Pattee, 1993; Bierman, Smoot, & Aumiller, 1993). Peer rejection directly increases aggressive behavior (Pettit, 1997) and hyperactive children are especially at risk of being rejected by peers (Satterfield & Schell, 1997). With the rise of the mega-schools, high schools with enrollments in the thousands, rejection may become commonplace as adolescent status competition becomes increasingly more intense.

Humans are social animals and children undergo the longest period of socialization of any animal, a dependency of two decades or longer. Intelligence, along with the disproportionately large neocortex of primates, may be an adaptation to the special complexities of primate social life (Byrne & Whitten, 1988), with the relative size of neocortex limiting the number of individuals a primate can significantly interact with on a regular basis (Dunbar, 1992). A so-called natural group size, when exceeded, is socially unstable and often results in social conflict and group splintering (Dunbar, 1993). If the natural group size of adult humans is approximately 150 individuals, as Dunbar (1993) has suggested, then it is irrational to expect children to develop normally in larger groups than they are biologically equipped to deal with. In a seminal study on social functioning and high school size, Barker and Gump (1964) determined that students in smaller schools participated in twice as many extracurricular activities as students in larger schools (grade size of 225 or more). Cotton (1996) reviewed 103 studies that investigated associations between high school size and factors such as academic performance, social behavior, dropout rate, and parental involvement, and concluded that smaller schools are beneficial to students in all domains of function regardless of rural or urban setting. Smaller schools were superior to larger schools on athletic participation, extracurricular activity participation, absenteeism, dropout rate, student satisfaction, minor and serious rule infractions, self-esteem and locus of control, interpersonal relationships, sense of community, parental involvement, interpersonal relations between teacher and students, and even teacher attitudes (Cotton, 1996). Compared to larger schools (enrollments above 600), smaller schools (400-600 enrollment) experience one-eighth the rate of serious crimes (4% compared to 33%), one-tenth the rate of physical attacks with weapons (2% to 20%), and one-third the rate of theft or larceny (18% to 68%) and vandalism (23% to 62%; Devoe et al., 2002). Academically, math and reading scores improved most for high school enrollments between 600 and 900 (Lee & Smith, 1997), with an even smaller optimum size (i.e., 450-650 enrollment) for mathematics achievement (based on their data scatter plot).

Small schools are more accountable to students and cost significantly less per graduate than larger schools (Stiefel, Latrola, Fruchter, & Berne, 1998). The National Association of Secondary School Principals (1996) recommended that secondary schools be capped at 600 students, and the Cross City Campaign for Urban School Reform recommended a limit of 500 students (Fine & Somerville, 1998). The existence of large schools is an outdated response to economic and social forces of the 1950s and 1960s. In 1959 and again in 1967 James Conant, past president of Harvard University, contended that the small high school was the number one problem in education and advocated for its elimination through district and school consolidation. In 1940, there were 200,000 public elementary and secondary schools, which have since been whittled down to less than a third of this number, 65,000 public elementary and secondary schools in 2005. Ironically this reduction occurred as the US population *increased* by 70 percent. Today some believe the number one problem in education is the large school (Quindlen, 2001).

School shootings are relatively rare, but may reflect systemic problems within educational institutions, ones that otherwise might be overlooked if not for such high-profile events. When the size of our schools exceeds the biocognitive capacity of our children, we are likely to witness fractures in a school's social fabric. Therefore it is hypothesized that a disproportionate amount of school shootings will take place in schools with grade size above our natural group size.

### *METHOD*

Seventeen cases of mass school shootings in public schools by students against students were examined between 1996 to 2005 as well as ten cases of post-Columbine averted school attacks. A school shooting is defined as an incident that took place on schools grounds, was committed by students of the school with clear lethal intent, and which resulted in multiple victimizations. Only one "school shooting" incident included in this analysis took place without the use of a firearm, when seven fellow students were injured by a machete and tree saw. Excluded from analysis are events perpetrated by adults, ex-students, or unknown assailants. Information about each school involved was acquired from the National Center for Educational Statistics (http://nces.ed.gov/ccd/) for the academic year of each incident, or estimated from the most recent complete data (academic year 2001-2002). Details were also taken from Stevens (2003), Newman, Fox, Harding, Mehta, and Roth (2004), National School Safety and Security Services (schoolsecurity.org), and media reports.

## RESULTS

As shown in Figure 1, 11 of 13 high school shootings took place where actual grade enrollment for the assailant(s) was greater than 150 students (Chi-square = 6.2, df = 1), $p < .05$. As brain maturation (and presumably associated social cognitive ability) is not complete until adulthood (age 18 or later), natural group size for immature brains was calculated using gray-to-white matter ratios recorded from Courchesne et al. (2001) in 52 normal children from age 2 to 16. Gray-white matter ratios decrease linearly with age as absolute and relative amounts of white matter increase with brain maturation (Courchesne et al., 2001). This recalculation of natural group size allows for further analysis of incidents perpetrated by younger children at the four middle school incidents. Table 1 presents gray-white matter ratios and adjusted natural group (or grade) size by age.

Fourteen of 17 school shootings took place in age-adjusted grade enrollments of more than 150 students (Chi-square = 7.1, df = 1), $p < .01$. Table 2 presents location, actual grade size, total injuries, and adjusted grade size for all incidents. Injuries per assailant correlated to a modest degree with grade size, $r = .40$, $t(15) = 1.67$, $p < .06$, and with adjusted grade size, $r = .41$, $t(15) = 1.73$, $p < .06$, as shown in Figure 2. No effect of grade size was found for post-Columbine averted school attacks (Chi-square = 1.6, df = 1), $p > .05$; see Table 3). Schools on the list of

FIGURE 1. Number of high school incidents by assailants' actual grade size since 1996.

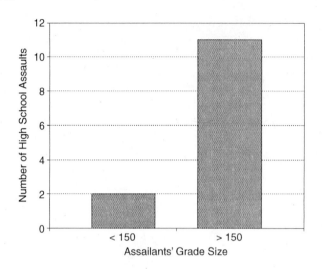

TABLE 1. Yearly Gray/White Matter Cortical Ratios Taken from Courchesne et al. (2001) and Subsequent Adjusted Maximum Natural Adolescent Group Size Assuming Adult Social Neurodevelopment by Age 18.

| Age in Years | 10 | 11 | 12 | 13 | 14 | 15 | 16 | 17[a] | 18[a] |
|---|---|---|---|---|---|---|---|---|---|
| G/W Ratio | 2.30 | 2.21 | 2.12 | 2.03 | 1.95 | 1.86 | 1.77 | 1.68 | 1.60 |
| Maximum Grade Size | 84 | 92 | 100 | 109 | 117 | 125 | 133 | 141 | 150 |

[a]Extrapolated ratios

averted attacks were selected without bias (i.e., without awareness of school size) from those reported in Newman et al. (2004) and schoolsecurity.org.

Public high school size was surveyed from the Common Core Data of the National Center for Educational Statistics for year 2000-2001. Median grade size in U.S. public high schools was 185 in the year 2000. Fifty-seven percent had enrollments above 150 students per grade. Compare this to 85 percent (11 of 13) of high school shootings that happened in schools with enrollments larger than 150 students per grade.

FIGURE 2. Injuries per assailant by age-adjusted grade size for middle and high school assaults.

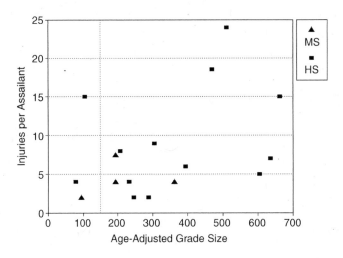

## *DISCUSSION*

In the past decade 17 high-profile school shootings occurred in public schools. Using census designations, seven shootings occurred in suburbs, four in towns, four in rural areas, and two in cities. Of 13 high school shootings, 7 involved total school enrollments of more than 1,000 students. Median high school grade size where a shooting took place was 272 compared to 185 in all public high schools. The correlation between injuries per assailant and grade size approached significance ($p < .06$), despite all the other possible factors that could influence attack severity including time of day, setting, marksmanship, assault duration, response of school security or police. This relationship between grade size and injuries may reflect the amount of planning, motivation, and determination on the part of assailants. Perhaps the larger the school, the greater the anonymity and the larger eventual response against its social structure.

Most of these attacks have been characterized as assaults against the adolescent social hierarchy (Newman et al., 2004). Schools are prime locations for socialization as well as victimization. Each year nearly 1 in 10 high school students report being bullied at school, and more report being threatened or injured with a weapon (DeVoe et al., 2004). Status

TABLE 2. Location, Grade Size (with and without age adjustment) and Total Injuries of Multiple Injury School Shootings from 1996 to 2005.

| Location | | Grade Size | Assailant Age(s) | Adj. Size | Total Injuries* |
|---|---|---|---|---|---|
| 6-8th grade | | | | | |
| Stamps | AR | 75 | 14 | 96 | 2 |
| Fort Gibson | OK | 141 | 13 | 194 | 4 |
| Jonesboro | AR | 120 | 11,13 | 194 | 15 |
| Edinboro | PA | 283 | 14 | 362 | 4 |
| | | | | | |
| 9th-12th grade | | | | | |
| Bethel | AK | 70 | 16 | 79 | 4 |
| Red Lake | MN | 95 | 16 | 107 | 15 |
| West Paducah | KY | 163 | 14 | 209 | 8 |
| Moses Lake | WA | 182 | 14 | 233 | 4 |
| Cold Spring | MN | 206 | 15 | 246 | 2 |
| Richmond | VA | 242 | 14 | 289 | 2 |
| Pearl | MS | 272 | 16 | 305 | 9 |
| Conyers | GA | 351 | 16 | 394 | 6 |
| Littleton | CO | 443 | 17,18 | 469 | 37 |
| Springfield | OR | 428 | 15 | 512 | 24 |
| El Cajon | CA | 604 | 18 | 604 | 5 |
| Valparaiso | IN | 532 | 15 | 636 | 7 |
| Santee | CA | 555 | 15 | 664 | 15 |

* includes fatalities

competition is fierce in crowded environments. When more than half of all public high schools exceed our natural group size, it is not surprising that abnormal and atypical social behaviors including violence frequently occur (see Table 4 for grade size as a function of locale). The process of socialization is likely prolonged and diminished in megaschools. Beside socialization, intellectual development is also likely to suffer in such large social settings as a great proportion of time and resources are spent maintaining an orderly learning environment at the expense of learning. Behavioral regulation through face-to-face interaction and rapport is beyond the capabilities of students, teachers, and administrators in larger schools, so formal institutions of security must be employed.

One hundred and fifty is said to be our species' natural group size, the size of groups that humans survived within for the vast majority of our history. In fact, one hundred and fifty individuals approximates the size

TABLE 3. Planned School Shootings 1999-2001.

| Location | Grade Size |
|----------|-----------:|
| Hoyt, KS | 67 |
| Mattawa, WA | 95 |
| Glendale, AZ | 97 |
| Port Huron, MI | 196 |
| Elmira, NY | 268 |
| Fort Collins, CO | 299 |
| Cleveland, OH | 392 |
| Carrollton, TX | 709 |
| New Bedford, MA | 820 |
| Santa Ana, CA | 1136 |

TABLE 4. Grade Size in Public High Schools as a Function of Locale.

| Locale | High Schools Number | Median Grade Size | Largest Size | Grade Size Above 150 |
|--------|--------------------:|------------------:|-------------:|---------------------:|
| City | 2,054 | 408 | 1,522 | 93% |
| Suburb | 3,.832 | 303 | 1,289 | 82% |
| Town | 2,175 | 159 | 745 | 53% |
| Rural | 4,980 | 86 | 1,244 | 25% |
| All Locales | 13,041 | 185 | 1,522 | 57% |

of many hunter-gatherer bands and horticultural villages today (Dunbar, 1993). When people are faced with a large number of faces (e.g., more than 150), their response has commonly been to leave, to separate. Bands and villages splinter into daughter groups and move apart when there are too many people to feed and figure out (i.e., when the group has become too complex for the tribe members' brain function; Dunbar, 1993). Humanity spread across the globe in a relatively short time in part because of the constant process of division down to appropriate-sized social groups. Children today, given the same chance to leave large numbers, will often take this option. As shown in Figure 3, ninth grade dropout rate correlated with grade size in mid-size cities and large towns (see Cotton, 2001 and Stiefel et al., 1998, for comparisons within cities). Too many faces lead to in-grouping and out-grouping, alienation and depression, cliques and conflicts. A school largely populated with strangers is an environment that children are biologically unsuited for,

FIGURE 3. Dropout rate for 9th graders of mid-size cities (locale 2) as a function of grade size (modified from Kaiser, 2002).

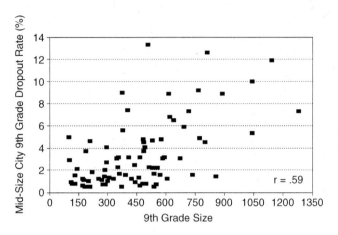

and from which many will retreat, emotionally if they cannot physically.

The assumption that social-related neurodevelopment is completed by 18 years of age is unlikely given post-adolescent brain growth in dorsolateral frontal cortex and other critical brain areas (Sowell, Thompson, Tessner, & Toga, 2001). Quantitative evidence of reduced functional coordination between anterior sites, presumably due to delayed or recent myelination, was found for 9 of 10 college-aged students (Kaiser, unpublished data, April 2005; see Figure 4). Perhaps optimal grade size should be adjusted accordingly even at the college level.

More and more educational and advocacy groups recognize that smaller schools serve our children best. As mentioned above, some have recommended a 600 enrollment limit based on practice and empirical evaluations (e.g., National Association of Secondary School Principals, 1996). This article reviewed literature on brain damage/dysfunction and social competition as factors in school violence, and provided evidence for a biological explanation for optimal school size (i.e., a neurobiological constraint on social relations). Adjusting to larger groups may tax neurocognitive functioning beyond the capabilities of many children. This may be especially true of right hemisphere-related functions such as empathy and other social skills. However, other factors obviously must be considered in cases of school shootings and violence. Recently a 16-year-old boy shot five classmates in a very small school

FIGURE 4. A representative college student's eyes closed comodulation data compared to adult norms. Comodulation is a measure of magnitude consistency between electrode pairs across time. Low magnitude consistency (colored blue, 2 standard deviations below the mean) indicates lower functional connectivity or coordination relative to an adult norm whereas green coloration reflects normal levels of comodulation. Each topograph represents a site compared to all other sites including itself (i.e., 19 pair-wise comparisons).

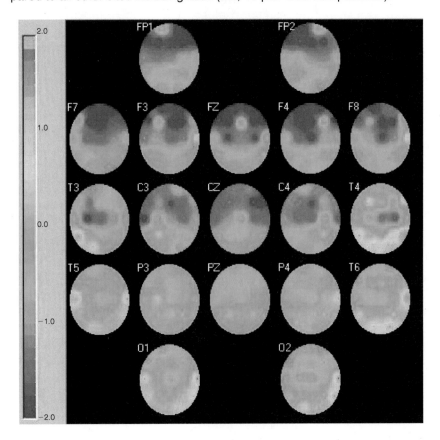

in Minnesota; clearly not all pressures faced by adolescents can be indexed by the size of the academic environment.

Reducing school size to within children's neurobiological capabilities is a universal prevention, a proactive method of reducing violence and improving intellectual, emotional, and social development. When groups are small enough for members to know one another, they are more apt and able to police themselves. When natural group sizes are exceeded, formal institutions of behavioral control are necessary, which can be both expensive and ineffective. Some communities have experimented with a schools-within-a-school approach, dividing large student bodies into smaller operational units with dedicated academic and administrative personnel. But common areas (gym, cafeteria, entrance) often remain shared by the entire student body, undermining group cohesion, and students in physically large schools rarely possess the freedoms and responsibilities of students in smaller schools, regardless of administrative strategy. We need to build smaller schools, more schools, and roll back the consolidation of the past half century. Realistically, excessively large schools will continue to be built and there will be children with acquired or inherited brain damage or dysfunction lacking in behavioral control and prone to violence in any size group. Selected and indicated prevention of violence in such individuals will require other approaches. Effective medications for attention deficit disorder, anxiety, depression, and seizure disorders exist and can be useful for many appropriately diagnosed children. In many cases such disorders co-exist in children with histories of violence. However, all have side effects, and often do not directly impact the specific brain systems underlying the type of behavioral dyscontrol involved in violent behaviors. A promising approach to prevention of violence in such at-risk children is neurotherapy (EEG biofeedback). This technique enables self-regulation of the bioelectrical functioning of the central nervous system, has few if any significant side effects, and has been demonstrated through research and extensive clinical use to be effective not only in control of co-existing disorders such as attention deficit disorder, but also in cases of episodic violence (Quirk, 1995). Nevertheless, while neurotherapy may improve an individual's behavior by normalizing brain activity, similar normalization of his or her social environment also seems essential.

## REFERENCES

Barker, R., & Gump, P. V. (1964). *Big school, small school.* Palo Alto, CA: Stanford University Press.

Bassarath, L. (2001). Neuroimaging studies of antisocial behaviour. *Canadian Journal of Psychiatry, 46,* 728-732.

Bierman, K. L., Smoot, D. L., & Aumiller, K. (1993). Characteristics of aggressive-rejected, aggressive (nonrejected), and rejected (nonaggressive) boys. *Child Development, 64,* 139-151.

Blair, R. J., & Cipolotti, L. (2000). Impaired social response reversal. A case of "acquired sociopathy." *Brain, 123,* 1122-1141.

Bradshaw, C. P., & Garbarino, J. (2004). Social cognition as a mediator of the influence of family and community violence on adolescent development: Implications for intervention. *Annals of the New York Academy of Sciences, 1036,* 85-105.

Byrne, R. W., & Whitten, A. (1988). *Machiavellian intelligence: Social expertise and the evolution of intellect in monkeys, apes and humans.* New York: Clarendon Press.

Conant, J. B. (1959). *The American high school today: A first report to interested citizens.* New York: McGraw-Hill.

Conant, J. B. (1967). *The comprehensive high school: A second report to interested citizens.* New York: McGraw-Hill.

Convit, A., Czobor, P., & Volavka, J. (1991). Lateralized abnormality in the EEG of persistently violent psychiatric inpatients. *Biological Psychiatry, 30,* 363-370.

Cotton, K. (1996). Affective and social benefits of small-scale schooling. Charleston, WV: Clearinghouse on Rural Education and Small Schools. (ERIC Document Reproduction Service No. ED401088).

Cotton, K. (2001). New small learning communities: Findings from recent literature. Portland, OR: Northwest Regional Educational Laboratory.

Courchesne, E., Karns, C. M., Davis, H. R., Ziccardi, R., Carper, R. A., Tigue, Z. D., et al. (2001). Unusual brain growth patterns in early life in patients with autistic disorder: An MRI study. *Neurology, 57,* 245-254.

Deckel, A. W., Hesselbrock, V., & Bauer, L. (1996). Antisocial personality disorder, childhood delinquency, and frontal brain functioning: EEG and neuropsychological findings. *Journal of Clinical Psychology, 52,* 639-650.

DeVoe, J. F., Peter, K., Kaufman, P., Ruddy, S. A., Miller, A. K., Planty, M., et al. (2002). Indicators of school crime and safety (NCES 2003-009/NCJ 196753). Washington DC: U.S. Departments of Education and Justice.

DeVoe, J. F., Peter, K., Kaufman, P., Miller A., Noonan, M., Snyder, T. D., et al. (2004). Indicators of school crime and safety (NCJ 205290). Washington DC: U.S. Departments of Education and Justice.

Dodge, K. A., Pettit, G. S., McClaskey, C. L., & Brown, M. (1986). Social competence in children. *Monographs of the Society for Research in Child Development,* 51, (2, Serial No. 213).

Dunbar, R. I. M. (1992). Neocortex size as a constraint on group size in primates. *Journal of Human Evolution, 20,* 469- 493.

Dunbar, R. I. M. (1993). Coevolution of neocortical size, group size and language in humans, *Behavioral and Brain Sciences, 16,* 681-735.

Evans, J. R., & Claycomb, S. (1999). Abnormal QEEG patterns associated with dissociation and violence. *Journal of Neurotherapy, 3* (2), 21-27.

Evans, J. R., & Park, N. (1997). Quantitative EEG findings among men convicted of murder. *Journal of Neurotherapy, 2* (2), 31-39.

Fine, M., & Somerville, J. I. (1998). Essential elements of small schools. In M. Fine & J. I. Somerville (Eds.), *Small schools, big imaginations: A creative look at urban public schools* (pp. 104-112). Chicago, IL: Cross City Campaign for Urban School Reform.

Kaiser, D. A. (2002, February). Preventing another Columbine: Natural group size of humans and what it means to secondary education. Paper presented at the 10th Annual Winter Brain Conference, Miami, FL.

Lee, V. E., & Smith, J. B. (1997). High school size: Which works best and for whom? *Educational Evaluation and Policy Analysis, 19,* 205-228.

Mason, M. F., & Macrae, C. N. (2004). Categorizing and individuating others: The neural substrates of person perception. *Journal of Cognitive Neuroscience, 16,* 1785-1795.

Mendez, M. F., Chen, A. K., Shapira, J. S., & Miller, B. L. (2005). Acquired sociopathy and frontotemporal dementia. *Dementia and Geriatric Cognitive Disorders, 20,* 99-104.

Mosch, S. C., Max, J. E., & Tranel, D. (2005). A matched lesion analysis of childhood versus adult-onset brain injury due to unilateral stroke: Another perspective on neural plasticity and recovery of social functioning. *Cognitive and Behavioral Neurology, 18,* 5-17.

Mychack, P., Kramer, J. H., Boone, K. B., & Miller, B. L. (2001). The influence of right frontotemporal dysfunction on social behavior in frontotemporal dementia. *Neurology, 56,* S11-S15.

National Association of Secondary School Principals (1996). *Breaking ranks: Changing an American institution.* A Report of the National Association of Secondary School Principals in partnership with the Carnegie Foundation for the Advancement of Teaching on the high school of the 21st century. Reston, VA: National Association of Secondary School Principals and Carnegie Foundation for the Advancement of Teaching.

Newcomb, A. F., Bukowski, W. M., & Pattee, L. (1993). Children's peer relations: A meta-analytic review of popular, rejected, neglected, controversial, and average sociometric status. *Psychological Bulletin, 113,* 99-128.

Newman, K. S., Fox, C., Harding, D. J., Mehta, J., & Roth, W. (2004*). Rampage: The social roots of school shootings.* New York: Basic Books.

Pettit, G. S. (1997). The developmental course of violence and aggression. *Psychiatric Clinics of North America, 20,* 283-299.

Quindlen, A. (2001, March 26). The problem of the megaschool. *Newsweek,* 68.

Quirk, D. A. (1995). Composite biofeedback conditioning and dangerous offenders: III. *Journal of Neurotherapy, 1* (2), 44-54

Satterfield, J. H., & Schell, A. M. (1997). A prospective study of hyperactive boys with conduct problems and normal boys: Adolescent and adult criminality. *Journal of the American Academy of Child Psychiatry, 36,* 1726-1735.

Silver, H., Goodman, C., Knoll, G., Isakov, V., & Modai, I. (2005). Schizophrenia patients with a history of severe violence differ from nonviolent schizophrenia patients in perception of emotions but not cognitive function. *Journal of Clinical Psychiatry, 66,* 300-308.

Sowell, E. R., Thompson, P. M., Tessner, K. D., & Toga, A. W. (2001). Mapping continued brain growth and gray matter density reduction in dorsal frontal cortex: Inverse relationships during post adolescent brain maturation. *Journal of Neuroscience, 21,* 8819-8829.

Stanton, B., Baldwin, R. M., & Rachuba, L. (1997). A quarter century of violence in the United States. An epidemiologic assessment. *Psychiatric Clinics of North America, 20,* 269-282.

Sterzer, P., Stadler, C., Krebs, A., Kleinschmidt, A., & Poustka, F. (2005). Abnormal neural responses to emotional visual stimuli in adolescents with conduct disorder. *Biological Psychiatry, 57,* 7-15.

Stevens, R. D. (2003). The National School Safety Center's Report on School-Associated Violent Death. Westlake Village, CA: National School Safety Center.

Stiefel, L., Latrola, P., Fruchter, N. A., & Berne, R. (1998). The effects of size of student body on school costs and performance in NYC high schools. New York: Institute for Education and Social Policy.

Tranel, D., Bechara, A., & Denburg, N. L. (2002). Asymmetric functional roles of right and left ventromedial prefrontal cortices in social conduct, decision-making, and emotional processing. *Cortex, 38,* 589-612.

Wrangham, R. W., & Wilson, M. L. (2004). Collective violence: Comparisons between youths and chimpanzees. *Annals of New York Academy of Sciences, 1036,* 233-256.

# Index

# BOOK ORDER FORM!

Order a copy of this book with this form or online at:
http://www.haworthpress.com/store/product.asp?sku= 5878

## Forensic Applications of QEEG and Neurotherapy

___ in softbound at $17.95 ISBN-13: 978-0-7890-3079-5 / ISBN-10: 0-7890-3079-9.
___ in hardbound at $34.95 ISBN-13: 978-0-7890-3078-8 / ISBN-10: 0-7890-3078-0.

| | |
|---|---|
| **COST OF BOOKS** _____ | ❑**BILL ME LATER:** |
| | Bill-me option is good on US/Canada/ |
| **POSTAGE & HANDLING** _____ | Mexico orders only; not good to jobbers, |
| US: $4.00 for first book & $1.50 | wholesalers, or subscription agencies. |
| for each additional book | |
| Outside US: $5.00 for first book | ❑**Signature** _____ |
| & $2.00 for each additional book. | |
| | **Payment Enclosed: $** _____ |
| **SUBTOTAL** _____ | |
| In Canada: add 7% GST._____ | ❑ **PLEASE CHARGE TO MY CREDIT CARD:** |
| | ❑Visa ❑MasterCard ❑AmEx ❑Discover |
| **STATE TAX** _____ | ❑Diner's Club ❑Eurocard ❑JCB |
| CA, IL, IN, MN, NJ, NY, OH, PA & SD residents | **Account #**_____ |
| please add appropriate local sales tax. | |
| | **Exp Date** _____ |
| **FINAL TOTAL** _____ | |
| If paying in Canadian funds, convert | **Signature** _____ |
| using the current exchange rate, | (Prices in US dollars and subject to change without notice.) |
| UNESCO coupons welcome. | |

PLEASE PRINT ALL INFORMATION OR ATTACH YOUR BUSINESS CARD

Name

Address

City          State/Province          Zip/Postal Code


Country

Tel          Fax

May we use your e-mail address for confirmations and other types of information? ❑Yes ❑No We appreciate receiving your e-mail address. Haworth would like to e-mail special discount offers to you, as a preferred customer.
**We will never share, rent, or exchange your e-mail address.** We regard such actions as an invasion of your privacy.

Order from your **local bookstore** or directly from
**The Haworth Press, Inc.** 10 Alice Street, Binghamton, New York 13904-1580 • USA
Call our toll-free number (1-800-429-6784) / Outside US/Canada: (607) 722-5857
Fax: 1-800-895-0582 / Outside US/Canada: (607) 771-0012
E-mail your order to us: orders@haworthpress.com

**For orders outside US and Canada,** you may wish to order through your local
sales representative, distributor, or bookseller.
For information, see http://haworthpress.com/distributors

(Discounts are available for individual orders in US and Canada only, not booksellers/distributors.)

**Please photocopy this form for your personal use.**
www.HaworthPress.com

BOF06